D1608864

# Second Spring

## A Guide to Healthy Menopause Through Traditional Chinese Medicine

by

## Honora Lee Wolfe

**Blue Poppy Press**

Published by:

**BLUE POPPY PRESS**
**1775 LINDEN AVE.**
**BOULDER, CO 80304**

**FIRST EDITION**
**OCTOBER 1990**

**ISBN 0-936185-18-X**

Printed at Westview Press, Boulder, CO
Cover printed at D & K Printing, Boulder, CO

This book is printed on archive quality, acid free, recycled paper.

# ACKNOWLEDGMENTS

Our decision at Blue Poppy Press to publish a book for laywomen about menopause was made over two years ago, but at that time it was not decided who on the Blue Poppy staff should write it. With the success of my previous book, *The Breast Connection,* I was urged by my husband, Bob Flaws, to take on this project. On the other hand, Bob is chief editor of Blue Poppy, and he had very specific ideas about a book on menopause and what it should contain. Additionally, he has much more experience than I have in the area of Traditional Chinese gynecology and Chinese medical theory in general. Bob's solid theoretical knowledge and previous research on menopause were invaluable to me and have greatly improved the clarity and thoroughness of the information presented here. Furthermore, his research on the Chinese energetic descriptions of vitamins and minerals which is included in Chapter Nine is ground breaking material not previously published anywhere. If readers find this book useful, they should know that it would not have been what it is without the help of Bob Flaws. It is his book at least as much as it is mine.

Honora Lee Wolfe
September, 1990

# TABLE OF CONTENTS

# INTRODUCTION

Menopause is a popular topic these days. Magazine articles and books abound on the subject. As the first women of the baby boom generation approach and enter this passage, they are demanding more information, new and better options for medical treatment when necessary, and alternatives to standard Western medical therapies. Also, the women who are now in their 40's and 50's were and are some of the first movers and shakers of the women's movement in the 1960's and 70's. We are, as a group, quite vocal, and not likely to traverse any important passage in our lives without it being well documented.

As I pass through my early 40's, the subject of menopause comes more often to my mind. As a practitioner of acupuncture, I see more and more women in the midst of this time in their lives. All those magazine articles, which 5 years ago I'd have barely skimmed if I'd have read them at all, seem to jump out of the table of contents and demand my attention. The impending loss of fertility and increasing reminders of aging in the mirror can no longer be ignored.

Whether or not we have come to terms with aging, mortality, or our existential dilemma, I and all my baby boom sisters must pass through menopause within the next decade or so. Typical

1

of my generation, I want this coming life passage to be as free as possible from despair, confusion, loss of self-esteem, and physical discomfort. Of course I may not get my way, but my assumption is that other women have similar feelings, and it is because of this assumption that I add yet another to the list of books on menopause.

There are many fine books available on menopause and related topics, several of which I have listed in the Suggested Reading list at the back. This book, however, is the only one (so far as I am aware) which discusses menopause entirely from the point of view of Traditional Chinese Medicine (TCM). I truly believe that TCM, its theories and its various therapies have a great deal to offer the menopausal woman. This book is designed to help women understand the theories of TCM vis-a-vis menopause, and to decide if TCM may help ease the possible physical and emotional discomforts which sometimes attend it.

Secondly, this book is about the prevention of the symptoms of what is called menopausal syndrome. Offered herein are a number of self-help ideas and disciplines to reduce stress, create purpose and self-esteem, and improve quality of life during menopause, or at any other time which is emotionally or physically trying.

Finally, this book is my own attempt to come to terms with approaching menopause and aging, and to document and share a part of that process with my readers. I wish us all good luck and good health.

# CHAPTER ONE
# THE WESTERN MEDICAL DESCRIPTION OF MENOPAUSE AND MENOPAUSAL SYNDROME

According to modern Western medicine, **natural menopause** is described as the transitional phase of a woman's life when menstrual function ceases due to age-related declining ovarian function usually occurring between the ages of 40 and 50. Around the end of the fourth or beginning of the fifth decade of life, a woman's ovaries cease producing estrogen and progesterone despite hormonal stimulation from the pituitary gland. Ovulation becomes less and less frequent and eventually stops. Estrogen blood levels fall below the point necessary to produce uterine bleeding so that periods slowly cease. Estrogen levels continue to decline slowly over another year or so until no estrogen at all is secreted from the ovaries.

It seems that it takes a while for the pituitary to get the message that the ovaries are no longer functioning. It continues to produce follicle stimulating hormone (FSH) and luteinizing hormone (LH) at high levels to try to get the ovaries to respond. The levels of these two hormones in the bloodstream becomes elevated at the time of menopause, while estrogen and progesterone levels are falling.

3

Although no longer secreted by the ovaries, estrogen is still being produced in the body, but in a slightly different form called estrone. It is manufactured by the body's fat cells from a precursor hormone called androstenedione, which is largely produced by the adrenal glands. This is one possible reason why some menopausal women put on weight, in the body's attempt to produce enough estrogen.[1]

According to Western medicine, early or **premature menopause**, or menopause prior to age 40, may occur for a variety of reasons. The most common of these include response to viral infection, inherited chromosomal abnormality, defects in gonadotropin secretion, autoimmune disorders, enzymatic defects, excessive smoking, or cancerous growths.[2]

**Artificial menopause** automatically follows the surgical removal of the ovaries, irradiation of the ovaries, or radium implants in the uterus, thus destroying them and their ability to secrete estrogen.[3]

Although the transition of menopause may occur without symptoms, at least 75% of women experience the most common menopausal symptoms -- hot flashes.[4] According to modern Western medicine, these are due to instability of the brain's relay system, its neurotransmitters, which are affected by the lowered levels of estrogen in the blood stream as menopause progresses. This instability affects our autonomic nervous system (ANS). It is the ANS which is responsible for our body's thermostatic control, contraction and dilation of the blood vessels and skin pores, perspiration, and other automatic physiological responses of our body. Another way to think about the ANS is that it is responsible for all the many things which go on in our bodies which are not usually within our conscious control.

4

It can take a while for this brain relay system to re-adjust itself to a new level of blood estrogen. For the average woman this usually means about a year of hot flashes, although some women experience them for much shorter or longer periods of time and some not at all.

A related problem is night sweats, which are really only hot flashes experienced at night. These are often more problematic than hot flashes during the day because they can disturb a woman's sleep, thereby causing other kinds of problems. In fact, some sources feel that the fatigue, irritability, and insomnia which some menopausal women report are merely side effects of frequent night-time hot flashes.[5]

Another common symptom of menopause is irregular periods with extremely heavy bleeding. Again, this seems to be related to the erratic brain relay system and lack of ovulation which results in irregular levels of estrogen in relationship to progesterone. Fibroid tumors, endometriosis, and uterine cancer are also possible causes. Excessive stress can make this problem worse. Excessive menopausal or postmenopausal bleeding is usually treated with estrogen replacement therapy (ERT), birth control pills, D & C, or, in extreme cases, hysterectomy.

Other symptoms which can effect women during menopause include depression, palpitations, numbness and tingling in the limbs, urinary frequency or incontinence, back pain, vaginal dryness or irritation, and various gastrointestinal disorders.[6]

Sometimes Western medical practitioners will look for an organic dysfunction responsible for these difficulties, such as high blood pressure and thyroid or pituitary disorders. Most often, however, the medical texts counsel the doctor to try and evaluate how many of these symptoms are psychogenic in origin.[7] In other words, modern Western medicine often tends to dismiss these problems as psychological or emotionally induced. This is because modern Western medicine posits no clear etiology or cause for these signs and symptoms.

Because Western medicine essentially defines menopausal problems as a lack of estrogen production, the main Western therapy prescribed for menopausal women is estrogen replacement therapy (ERT). The pros and cons of ERT are discussed in Appendix I of this book as well as in many other books on menopause. While not a panacea for the symptoms of aging, ERT can diminish or eliminate many of the troublesome symptoms of menopausal syndrome at least for a while. Especially hot flashes, night sweats, and joint or back pain due to bone decalcification will be positively affected by ERT. ERT also seems to have a positive effect on the elasticity of the arteries, thereby reducing the risk of heart disease.[8] Estrogen creams are also used locally to reverse vaginal inflammation and sensitivity as well as some cases of urinary incontinence.

ERT therapy, however, does have risks. It has been implicated as a factor in certain types of breast cancer. It is also linked to higher rates of endometrial cancer (cancer of the uterine lining). However, preliminary research indicates that the use of lower does of estrogen with progesterone added for part of the month reduce or negate this latter risk.[9] Additionally, ERT is usually not prescribed for women who smoke due to the possible increased risk in these women for blood clots and stroke. Finally, some women will have to discontinue ERT due to excess vaginal bleeding, sore breasts, nausea and vomiting, uterine cramps, or abdominal bloating. [10]

6

Other therapies which are sometimes prescribed for menopausal women can include androgens or males sex hormones for loss of sexual desire, thyroid hormones for boosting energy, anti-depressants for severe depression, psychotherapy and mild sedatives for irritability, anxiety, or sleep disturbances, and large doses of calcium to protect against progressive osteoporosis. Biofeedback therapy is sometimes recommended to help regulate and control ANS responses for improving hot flash symptoms.

Other problems may occur after menopause including post-menopausal bleeding, serious bone decalcification (osteoporosis), and increased incidence of heart disease. These problems will be discussed later in the sections on Chinese medical theories relating to menopause, preventive therapies professional treatments, and Appendix I and II.

I have not gone into great detail concerning Western medicine and menopausal syndrome. This is because there are few satisfactory treatments available for menopausal syndrome in Western medicine. Traditional Chinese Medicine (TCM), on the other hand, has a lot of safe and effective treatments for menopausal complaints and much wisdom concerning the whys and wherefores of these complaints. It is this information that I would like to share with American women. There are many other good books available which do discuss Western medicine and menopausal physiology quite completely. I refer the reader to these for more detail in the area of Western medicine and its research or knowledge on the subject of menopause. (See the Suggested Reading section in the back of this book.)

# CHAPTER TWO
# WHY CHOOSE TRADITIONAL CHINESE MEDICINE?

Chinese medicine has at least 2000 years of recorded clinical history and within that time many styles of medical practice have been developed. Since the Chinese communist revolution in 1949 the government of China has supported one particular style of Chinese medicine, which is called Traditional Chinese Medicine (TCM). In the last two decades, many Westerners have gone to China to study TCM, and it has become the dominant style of Chinese medicine taught and practiced in the U.S. with over 25 schools, a national school accrediting body, and a national board examination to test for minimum competency. Practitioners of TCM in the U.S. may have training in acupuncture, herbal medicine, massage, and/or a few other related modalities. When I use the term Chinese medicine in this book, I am referring to TCM.

There are many reasons why TCM is a good choice for women with gynecological problems, menopausal syndrome included. I'll try to outline them as succinctly as possible.

## CHINESE MEDICINE IS HOLISTIC

First, Chinese medicine is one of the most holistic medical systems available today. This manifests in a number of ways. One example is that it does not segment health problems as either physical or psychological entities. One of the most enlightened aspects of Chinese medicine is that it never created a mind/body dualism. To think that one does not affect the other is absurd. To a practitioner of TCM, an emotional or mental event or experience is only another piece of diagnostic information, no different or less important that a physical sign or symptom. Treatment plans using acupuncture or herbal medicine typically include certain emotional tendencies or experiences as part of the overall pattern of disharmony being treated. While some practitioners of Chinese medicine may suggest the support of psychotherapy, just as many others may feel that acupuncture treatment is often as effective a method of working with certain emotional states. Classically, Chinese medical theory expects specific mental/emotional conditions to go along with certain disease patterns, and expects these emotional symptoms to respond to treatment as well as any physical symptom.

Further, in Chinese medicine each and every sign and symptom is only understood or interpreted in relationship to all the others. For example, a woman may come to a practitioner with complaints such as lower abdominal gas and bloating, loose bowel movements, appetite fluctuations, premenstrual symptoms such as irritability and breast tenderness, dizziness, fatigue, and low back pain. The Western medical practitioner might prescribe one medicine for the loose bowels, another for the appetite fluctuations, another for the PMS irritability, another for the back pain, and yet another for the dizziness. Furthermore, the MD might choose to send the patient to two or three specialists - an internist or gastro-enterologist for the digestive problems, a gynecologist for the PMS symptoms, an orthopedist for the back pain, a neurologist for the dizziness.

On the other hand, a good practitioner of Traditional Chinese Medicine sees and understands the *whole pattern* of this patient

10

as if she were a landscape painting with various aspects - water, trees, mountains, etc. - but all of one piece. The practitioner then prescribes singly or a combination of acupuncture, herbal, nutritional, exercise, and/or massage therapies to work effectively with the entire pattern that that patient presents. Done skillfully, Chinese medicine need not, indeed cannot, separate a person into segmented parts treating one symptom or part at the expense of another. Each part is only relevant in relationship to the whole of each patient's personal "landscape". Further, any change of even one sign or symptom may change the entire pattern, and therefore the entire treatment plan. In this way Traditional Chinese Medicine is indeed a holistic and humane system of medicine.

# CHINESE MEDICINE IS INDIVIDUALIZED

The second reason why a person might consider the use of Chinese medicine is that, because of its holistic view, it is more specific for each patient's needs than is Western medicine. A good example of this is the treatment of the Western named disease diabetes. The basic Western prescription for diabetes is insulin, which comes in several forms. These largely work on the principle of preventing hyperglycemia and glucosuria (elevated sugar in the blood and urine). This in turn helps minimize the damage to blood vessels and nervous tissue associated with severe cases of diabetes, and prevents insulin shock.[11] In Chinese medicine, however, a person with a Western diagnosis of diabetes must still go through a complete TCM diagnosis. This diagnosis can reveal any one of five or six simple patterns and a myriad of individualized complex patterns of disharmony which can account for a specific person's diabetes. Each of these patterns requires a different kind of treatment from the others, making it more specific to

11

that particular person's needs and imbalance. lessening the possibility for that person to experience Such personally tailored treatment lessens the possibility of that person experiencing unnecessary side effects.

# CHINESE MEDICINE HAS NO SIDE EFFECTS

The third reason for choosing Traditional Chinese medicine is that it is non-iatrogenic. That is to say, if the diagnosis has been correct, the treatments prescribed by Chinese medicine have no side effects. Although some side-effects initially may be experienced with herbal medicines, they are usually mild, and can be corrected by adjustments in the herbal formula. Acupuncture rarely has unwanted side-effects. Occasionally a client will report being excessively drowsy for a few hours after a treatment, or mild numbness or aching at one or another site of needle insertion, but long term or debilitating side effects are unknown. Even if the desired therapeutic effect vis a vis the major complaint is not achieved, most patients report feeling relaxed and comfortable after a treatment. For most people seeking Chinese medical help no negative side effects are experienced. In contradistinction, most drugs listed in a *Physician's Desk Reference (PDR)* have at least some expected and normal side effects and many have potentially serious irreversible side effects.

# CHINESE MEDICINE IS PREVENTIVE MEDICINE

Another reason why TCM is a good choice for women is because it is energetic medicine as well as or even more than material medicine. To understand the importance of this we must again use a comparison to Western medicine. Western

12

medical science is based on a reductionist material model of reality. This means that Western medicine mostly understands disease mechanisms by identifying and measuring smaller and smaller particles of matter and then manipulating those particles through drug therapy or removing sections of matter from within the body. Treatment can only be given if there is a measurable or quantifiable change in some bodily tissue or substance. This means Western medical treatment can be given only after disease has already progressed to the point of creating a quantifiable material change in the body.

Chinese medicine, by contrast, is energetic and functional in its orientation. The theories of Chinese medicine show us that often before any *measurable* change can occur in the tissues of the body, there will be energetic or functional changes which the patient will experience subjectively. Persons may complain of having a lump in the throat or sighing all the time, of feeling inappropriate anger or feeling that their lower body is cold as ice, or that they have feeling of anxious emptiness in their heart. To the Western MD, none of these symptoms may be clinically useful, yet blood or other tissue samples may also reveal nothing of clinical value. The person may have what Western medicine calls a purely functional disorder. The patient may clearly feel dis-eased, but the Western doctor may not be able to make a diagnosis. To the practitioner of TCM, however, these types of symptoms have great clinical meaning. They indicate to him or her that energetic changes have occurred in the body/mind which, if untreated over a period of time, will lead to tissue changes, and therefore more serious diseases.

This is significant because it means that a good practitioner of TCM can treat disease at a more fundamental level which then helps prevent the arisal of more serious disease. Therefore,

Chinese medicine is good preventive medicine, as well as being able to treat signs and symptoms which Western medicine sees as subclinical and therefore does not recognize as disease. This is especially important in the treatment of gynecological disorders, so many of which involve functional, emotional, and from the Western medical point of view, often subclinical signs and symptoms.

# CHINESE MEDICINE'S HISTORY OF SUCCESS

Traditional Chinese medicine has a long history of clinical success. The literature recording and verifying this history extends back over 2000 years or more and includes over 30,000 volumes. By comparison, modern Western medicine as it has been practiced over the last 50-100 years is a very young system. Many of the newest Western medical treatments for a given ailment have yet to be tried over even one generation allowing determination or measurement of long term side effects. On the other hand, many Western medical treatments are quite wonderful and it is not my intention to say that we should dismiss this system entirely. Rather modern Western medicine might be best seen as part of a larger system of medicine which allows people more options, and more levels of response. At times the swift and heroic treatments of Western medicine are useful and necessary in serious, acute, or life-threatening situations. For chronic or functional disorders, however, Chinese medicine offers a viable alternative, indeed an effective and humane alternative in areas which Western medicine offers few options or only treatments with many uncomfortable and possibly dangerous side effects.

14

Gynecology in general is an area in which Chinese medicine shines. Its treatment is humane, without side effects, and relatively inexpensive for a wide variety of disorders. Furthermore, Chinese medical theories are based upon direct observation of nature, as opposed to the abstract, mathematical complexities of histology and biochemistry in Western medicine. It is easier for a patient to grasp an understanding of their disease and its process as seen and described by Chinese medical theory, and it is usually far more empowering. To tell a patient, for example, that she has abnormally shaped red blood cells, or an elevated white blood cell count suggesting the presence of a bacterial infection, which is treated by so many days or weeks of this or that drug, may not be meaningful and may not allow her an understanding or an entrance for working with her disorder herself.[12] On the other hand, a practitioner of TCM may, for example, tell a patient that her Liver and Stomach are overheated. This is due to congested energy rather like heat in a pressure cooker. This condition, the practitioner continues, is related largely to dietary factors and stress, and these can be controlled by limiting certain foods in the diet, and by controlling stress which is like turning off the fire underneath the pressure cooker. Acupuncture may help reroute the Heat or clear it from the Organs which it is affecting. Such patient education gives the client a metaphor for seeing her psychophysical process, logically leading to possible responses she can make to improve or control her own health. In this way Chinese medicine is immediately understandable and empowering for the client. Its explanations and metaphors describing the disease process come from the natural world, to which most people can easily relate. It is not conceptually distant and opaque.

To recapitulate, there are six reasons why a woman may want to consider Chinese medical treatment for a menopausal, or any other gynecological disorder. 1) It is holistic, describing and evaluating the whole landscape of the bodymind, each part and piece in relationship to the others. 2) As a medical system, it has no inherently dangerous or troublesome side effects. 3) Its diagnostic techniques allow for great precision in seeing each individual quite specifically and thereby creating treatment plans which are equally precise. 4) It is a medicine which is more effective at manipulating energy than matter, and sees energetic change in the body as more fundamental than material change. By treating energetic imbalance effectively, gross material or substantial disease need not arise. This means that Chinese medicine is a preventive system of medicine. 5) Chinese medicine has a long, clinically verified history of effective treatment for most types of disease, including gynecology. 6) It is an understandable and empowering system of medicine, allowing patients a chance to understand their disease process and thereby the chance to participate in their healing process.

# CHAPTER THREE
# CHINESE MEDICAL THEORIES PERTAINING TO MENOPAUSE

In order to understand the phenomenon of menopause from the point of view of Traditional Chinese Medicine (TCM), we first must understand the theories explaining menstruation, Organ function, the Emotions in relationship to the Organs, Yin and Yang, and the production, storage and circulation of Blood, Energy (*Qi*), Body Fluids, and Vital Essence (*Jing*). In this chapter we will try to break down these theories into simple parts which, when put back together, will allow the reader to understand what a doctor of TCM understands when he or she evaluates a patient with menopausal symptoms.

## THE MAP IS NOT THE TERRAIN

For the reader to understand these theories, she must, as much as possible, forget about Western medical science, biology, and physiology. Chinese medicine has its own complete and self-contained description of the body and its functions. Its theories of physiology cannot and should not be compared with Western medicine. I like to use the metaphor of different kinds of maps. There are rainfall maps, population maps, topographic maps, and road maps. Each is self-contained and logical according to its own criteria. Each is a description of one aspect of reality and each has a different use. This is also true of Chinese medicine and Western medicine. Each has its own logic, rationale, and self-consistent view of reality. But each is only one map - and the map is not the terrain. In our culture, Western medical science has come to be believed as somehow really REAL, instead of one possible view, one level of how things are. Neither view negates the other, but it is best not to try and mix or cross reference one to the other.

Another challenge in understanding Chinese medicine has to do with translation. Our language is linear, deductive, and denotative. Chinese is eliptical, inductive, and connotative. Yet we must use certain words to translate from the Chinese. In this book the most important words presenting translational difficulty have to do with body Organs and tissues. The word Blood is a good example of this problem. In Chinese medicine the Blood (*Xue*) means something more than just the red fluid which flows through the arteries and veins. It has to do with the function of nutrition and nurturance altogether. It is energetic as well as substantive. Therefore, once again, the reader must forget her notions of blood from the point of view of Western physiology in order to understand the Chinese concept of Blood.

This is also true for the various Chinese Organs, whose descriptions sometimes overlap with those of Western physiology, but are much broader, and conceptually quite different. Chinese Organs are described by energetic, not chemical, functions, and must be thought of as freshly as possible in the reader's mind. Unfortunately, we have no adequate words to use in our language and so must use the words we have. However, where a word is capitalized (e.g. Blood, Sinews, Liver, Fluids, etc.), the reader must set aside her old concepts of that word, and try as best she can to adopt a beginner's mind, allowing a new map of the body to come into focus.

# A WORD ABOUT YIN AND YANG

Yin and Yang are terms in Chinese philosophy and medicine used to describe the polarization of all phenomena in the universe. As such, a basic understanding of Yin and Yang is vital to understanding Chinese medicine. As a result of the constant flux and interplay of these two opposing forces, all things evolve and devolve.

In the West, these words have been bandied about in many erroneous ways, and there are many misconceptions as the their meaning. Let us try to present them as clearly as possible in relation to the body and to Chinese medicine.

1. Yin and Yang are generic concepts describing opposing aspects or phenomena in nature. They may represent any two opposing objects or concepts or opposite aspects within a single object.

2. In all situation, Yin and Yang are interdependent. One does not, cannot exist without the other, just as dark implies light. In opposition they create unity.

3. Their relationship is in constant flux within a living being or system, just as the seasons follow one upon the next. Although health is the relative balance of Yin and Yang, this is never a static balance.

4. In the human body or in nature two natural symbols guide the classification of all other phenomena into Yin and Yang categories. These are Fire and Water. Fire is Yang and

19

Water is Yin. Any object that has properties or causes energetic change similar to those of Fire or Water may be described similarly as predominately Yang or Yin.

5. Yin and Yang are only relative concepts. An object or phenomenon can be Yin in one situation or comparison, and Yang in another. They are not absolute/they imply no value judgment.

6. Within the body it is said that Qi (movement and function) is Yang in relation to Blood (substance and nourishment) and that *Jing* (primal substance) is Yin in relationship to Spirit (primal movement). Within the body Yin and Yang must remain in dynamic harmonious balance. Yang must quicken Yin; Yin must nourish, cool, and root Yang. Life requires them both, as the seed sprouts in Spring only with the nourishment of the soil and melting snow (Yin), and the warmth of the sun (Yang).

7. If the harmonious relationship of interpromotion and restraint is lost between Yin and Yang in the body or in nature, disorder and discomfort will arise. Again, this will be explained in greater detail in later chapters. The chart below gives some basic opposite aspects of physiology in relationship to Yin and Yang.

However, in looking at this chart, it is of utmost importance to remember that these Yin Yang dichotomies only describe the relationships between these givens. Darkness is Yin only in comparison to light. It in no way implies that females are dark or males are light or that females are cold and males are hot. Nothing is inherently Yin or Yang. Something is more Yin or Yang in relationship to something else. Ultimately, there is no thing that is Yin or Yang. Yin Yang theory is only a descriptive conceptualization.

| Yang | Yin |
| --- | --- |
| Heaven | Earth |
| Day | Night |
| Spring/Summer | Autumn/Winter |
| Male | Female |
| Hot | Cold |
| Light | Darkness |
| Light | Heavy |
| Upward/Outward | Downward/Inward |
| Surface | Bones |
| Bowels | Organs |
| Agitated | Calm |
| *Wei* Qi Level | Blood Level |

# VITAL SUBSTANCES
# QI, BLOOD, BODY FLUIDS, AND *JING*

As stated above, Chinese medical physiology is quite different from Western, and volumes have been written on it. Although such detail is not necessary in this case, a minimal understanding of a few key words and concepts will be helpful to the

21

reader. Four of the most important of these are Qi, Blood, Body Fluids, and *Jing*. These words are difficult if not impossible to translate, but we can get a basic idea by considering their functions.

## QI

This is perhaps the most difficult of these four words to describe. One English language writer has called Qi "energy on the verge of becoming matter, or matter on the verge of becoming energy."[13] Dr. Liang, director of one of the first colleges of acupuncture in the U.S. describes Qi as follows:

> The concept of Qi is unlimited. Any movement, regardles of how small or how large, how brief or how long, how quick of how slow is caused by Qi. When Qi concentrates it is called Matter, and where it spreads it is called Space. When Qi gathers together it is called life, and when it separates it is called death. When Qi flows it is called health and when it is blocked there is disease.
>
> Planets depend upon it for their brightness. Weather is formed by it. The seasons are caused by it. Man cannot stand outside of Qi. It supports him and permeates him as water is contained within the ocean. [14]

22

These are eloquent and poetic descriptions, which give some idea of the difficulty of translating so many Chinese medical terms. The simplest way to understand Qi, however, is that Qi is function (as compared to structure). It is Yang in relationship to Blood being Yin. In the body, all physiologic activity is described by and dependent upon the movements and mutations of Qi. The five basic functions or intrinsic characteristics of Qi are:

> Propulsion/movement: Qi propels the Blood, transports nutritive substance to the entire body, and circulates the Body Fluids.

> Warming: Qi maintains the body temperature and by its warming nature energizes all the functional activities of the organism.

> Defense: Qi defends the body Surface against invasion by Exogenous pathogens.

> Transformation: Qi transforms the Blood and Body Fluids. It creates these out of the raw materials derived from respiration and digestion.

> Restraint or Astringency: The Qi holds the Blood within its Vessels, the Body Fluids within the body, and the Organs up against gravity.

We will see later what happens when there is any breakdown in any of these functions.

## BLOOD (*XUE*)

Described as the substance which flows through the vessels, the main function of Blood is to nourish. It is more material, physical, or Yin than Qi. In the *Nei Jing*, one of Chinese medicine's first classics, it is said that "The Qi commands the Blood, the Blood is the Mother of the Qi". This statement describes the basic difference between Qi and Blood or the Yin Yang polarity between them. If Qi is responsible for movement, warmth, transformation, and restraint of the Blood, Blood is the underlying nourishment which allows the Qi these functions. Without Blood or nourishment (Yin) the Qi (Yang) has no root, no material or substantial foundation or mother. Without Qi (Yang) to move, warm, and transform the Blood (Yin), the Blood is inert, without force or direction. As always Yin and Yang are completely interdependent.

Another statement from the *Nei Jing Su Wen*, elucidates the function of Blood for us more fully.

> The Liver receives the Blood, so there is sight.
> The legs receive Blood, thus they are able to
> walk. The hands receive Blood and so are able
> to grip. The fingers receive Blood and are then

able to grasp.

The Blood is the nutritive substance which the Qi then consumes, transforms, evaporates to create function.

Blood also has a strong relationship to healthy psychological functioning which will be discussed in the section covering Organ functions and emotions. When there is adequate Blood to nourish each Organ, a person's emotions/Spirit will be calm.


## BODY FLUIDS

Also a part of the Yin of the body, the Body Fluids is a general terms for all normal water/fluids within the body. They themselves are also subdivided into Yin and Yang. The Yin are those thick viscous fluids which nourish the joints and internal Organs, and which cushion the brain and spinal cord. The Yang are the lighter, thinner fluids such as tears, saliva, sweat, urine, gastric juice, and interstitial fluid. The functions of the Body Fluids are to moisten the skin, hair, joints, Organs, and tissues of the body, and to facilitate smooth movement of joints and other body parts. Blood and Body Fluids are derived from a common source, and may affect each other, for instance, consumption of Blood may injure the Body Fluids, and vice versa.

It is the Qi which is responsible for the movement and trans-

25

formation of Body Fluids. Qi evaporates and disperses the Body Fluids to all parts of the body. Therefore, an insufficiency of Qi may result in Body Fluids accumulating somewhere in the body as pathogenic Dampness.


### *JING*, VITAL ESSENCE

*Jing* refers to the vital physical essence of the body, its seminal basis. It is the primary substantial element responsible for determining physical growth and development and maintenance of life activity and metabolism. It is the most primal stuff from which our being unfolds. The outward physical manifestation of *Jing* in women is (menstrual) Blood; in men it is semen. It is the material base necessary for the creation of a new being, the creation of life. Therefore *Jing* is Yin in relationship to Spirit, which is the non-material or Yang impetus necessary for the creation of life. As we will see below, in Chinese medicine there are two types of *Jing*, Pre and Postnatal. The relationship of *Jing* to Qi and Blood is somewhat complex, and due to its importance in relationship to menopause, this relationship deserves a section of its own.


## *JING*, QI, BLOOD, AND AGING

When a baby is conceived, it is endowed with a certain complement of Vital Essence or *Jing* from its parents, based

26

upon their constitutional vigor, age, and current health. This is called in Chinese medicine Prenatal *Jing*. This is one's constitutional inheritance and it cannot be augmented. When this supply is used up in the process of living, a person dies, very much like a candle which goes out when its wax is used up. This fact is central to understanding the importance of menopause as a homeostatic mechanism which slows down the aging process in women.

When a baby is born, it takes its first breath and suckles its first food. From that moment on it is responsible for the creation of its own Qi and Blood, which previously it received from its mother in utero. This is called the Postnatal production of Qi and Blood. When a person is young and healthy and their digestion strong, they typically produce an overabundance of Qi and Blood or more than their body needs to function and maintain health day to day. During sleep each night this surplus is transformed by the body into Postnatal or Acquired Essence or *Jing*. This is stored by the Kidneys, as if in a bank, for use in emergencies or if the production of Postnatal *Jing* falls off for any reason. As long as digestion is good and the body is not overtaxed or ill, there will be surplus production of Postnatal Qi and Blood, and therefore abundant Postnatal or Acquired *Jing*. This Postnatal *Jing* bolsters Prenatal *Jing* and slows down the consumption of that original endowment. It is rather like living on the interest from one's wise investments (good diet and healthy lifestyle producing plenty of Qi and Blood) so that one does not consume one's

27

initial capital (their Prenatal *Jing*).

In women this surplus of Qi and Blood which leads to production of Postnatal or Acquired *Jing* is directly related to the menses. From the point of view of Chinese medicine, menstruation is due to a superabundance of Blood produced by a healthy woman which brims over about every 28 days.

At around the age of 35-40, this production cycle begins to slow down with the natural process of aging. The digestion becomes less efficient, therefore producing less Qi and Blood. This is relevant to menopause for two interrelated reasons. First, it means that over time there is not the production of the superabundance of Blood required for menstruation. Second, it means that less Postnatal or Acquired *Jing* is available to supplement Prenatal *Jing*. This leads to the consumption of Prenatal *Jing* which describes the aging process.

One of the reasons why menopause is a necessary, vital homeostatic mechanism in women's bodies is that by ending the monthly loss of Blood the consumption of both Blood and Prenatal *Jing* is slowed down. This is because, as it is said in the classics, *Jing* and Blood share a common source, the Kidneys. When Blood is lost with the menses each month some *Jing* is also lost since menstrual Blood, as stated above, is the physical manifestation of *Jing* in women. As the body metabolism slows down and less Blood, Qi, and Postnatal *Jing* is created, the body can ill-afford the monthly loss of Blood

28

(and *Jing)* of menstruation. The body's wisdom slows and then stops the menstrual flow, allowing the body to hold onto the Blood and *Jing*, which are more precious, since less is being created.

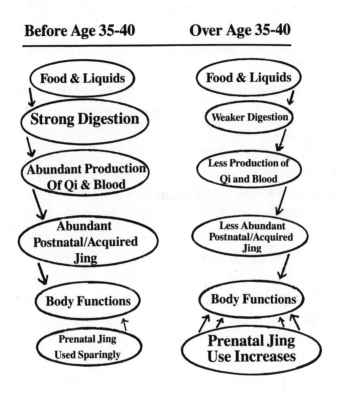

**Before Age 35-40**

Food & Liquids
Strong Digestion
Abundant Production Of Qi & Blood
Abundant Postnatal/Acquired Jing
Body Functions
Prenatal Jing Used Sparingly

**Over Age 35-40**

Food & Liquids
Weaker Digestion
Less Production of Qi and Blood
Less Abundant Postnatal/Acquired Jing
Body Functions
Prenatal Jing Use Increases

**Figure 1.**
**The Creation of Qi, Blood, and *Jing***
**In Relationship To Aging**

29

Thus, the menopause allows a woman the possibility for another 20 to 30 years of relative good health, with much slower decline than would be the case if menstruation continued. Menopause, while itself a sign of aging, actually slows down the aging process by preventing the unnecessary loss of Blood and *Jing*. Figure 1 gives a visual overview of the processes we have just gone over.

# ORGANS, CHANNELS, AND THE SEVEN EMOTIONS

Chinese medicine recognizes five Yin Organs and six Yang Bowels in the body. As stated in the introduction to this chapter, while there is some overlapping, the Chinese descriptions of these Organs and Bowels are very different from those of Western medical physiology. These differences are largely due to the fact that all descriptions of anything in TCM are energetic more than material. Chinese medicine is not much concerned with the chemical composition of cells or tissues within the Organs, or even with the gross physical structure of the Organs. Rather its emphasis is on what functions or energetic transformations in the body an Organ engenders, controls, promotes, or inhibits, and what happens or doesn't happen when an Organ is imbalanced or diseased.

In addition to being responsible for various internal transformations resulting in the creation and/or storage and release of pure substances (Qi, Blood, Body Fluids, *Jing*), each Organ is also responsible for the normal functioning of a particular layer of body tissue, a particular sensory ability, one of the five "spirits" or aspects of the psyche, and the expression of a particular emotion. (See Figure 2). This means that a Chinese Organ is not just a piece of differentiated tissue within the abdominal or thoracic cavity, but is a functional orb or a zone of greatly concentrated energetic activity within the overall energetic grid or circuitry of the body. Each Organ is an energy vortex and the sphere of influence of each Organ can and does extend to many other parts of the body, via pathways which Chinese medicine calls Channels and Collaterals.

| Organ | Tissue | Sense | Five Spirits | Emotion |
|---|---|---|---|---|
| Heart | Blood Vessels | Speech | Spirit/ Mind | Joy/ Fright |
| Spleen | Flesh | Taste | Thought/ Memory | Excessive Thinking/Worry |
| Lung | Skin/ Body Hair | Smell | Animal Vitality | Grief |
| Kidneys | Bones/ Head Hair | Hearing | Will Power | Fear |
| Liver | Jin/Sinews | Sight | Psyche/Ego | Anger |

**Figure 2.**
**Chinese Organs' Areas of Influence**

31

Channels and Collaterals, or what are more commonly referred to in the English language literature as Meridians, are sometimes described by Western authors as the electrical wiring of the body. They are the pathways over which the Qi flows, the routes by which the Organs and the various types of Qi manifest their functions and communicate with each other. These Channels and Collaterals are not visible conduits which can be seen upon dissection of the body, but their existence can be measured electrically and can also be felt by the propagation of acupuncture needle sensation along their pathways. The pathways of these Channels or Meridians are quite distinct, and have been well delineated in the Chinese medical literature for over two millennia. Current research suggests that these Meridians over which the Qi flows are the fascial planes in the connective tissue which bind the entire body together into one energetically connected unit.

Each Organ has its own related Channel, but the Meridian system as a whole forms one interconnected grid which functions as a sophisticated communication system. It is not within the scope of this book to describe in detail all the pathways of each Organ's Meridian or how they inter-relate, but in our discussion of specific symptoms in the following chapter, we will refer to certain Meridian routes to describe why certain symptoms appear in specific parts of the body. Readers interested in learning more about the Meridians are referred to the Suggested Reading section in the back for books on Chinese medicine which contain detailed descriptions of this Meridian system.

As stated above, each Organ is related to, or facilitates the expression of one or more emotion. The experience of any emotion is, from the Chinese medical point of view, merely the subjective experience of Qi flowing in specific directions in relationship to the normal directional flow of Qi in the related Organ. For example, the normal direction of flow of the Kidney Qi is inward or astringing. In moments of great fear, the Qi sinks or moves rapidly down. The physical experience of this sinking may be great urgency to urinate or a literal sinking feeling in the body as the Kidney Qi momentarily loses its astringent ability in response to the fear.

Normally, an emotion comes or "bubbles up" as it were, is experienced, and passes on based upon the organism's reaction to an appropriate stimuli. This is the normal, healthy experience of emotional states. If life situations cause one particular emotion to arise continually or to remain present for an unnatural length of time, (days, weeks, months, or years), this can cause imbalance in the Organ to which that emotion relates. Conversely, if an Organ is out of balance for any reason, this can lead to an imbalance in the experiencing of the emotion connected to that Organ. This can become a vicous cicle, where the emotion further imbalances an already out of balance Organ, leading to more experience of the emotion, and further imbalance of the Organ. We will discuss this in further detail in the next chapter under irritability and depression.

# THE ENDOCRINE SYSTEM AND CHINESE MEDICINE

Another notable difference between Chinese and Western physiology is the fact that traditional Chinese medicine does not recognize a separate endocrine system, nor does it describe any endocrine glands. This is not to say that traditional Chinese doctors do not take into account the functions of the endocrine system. They do. Nor it is to say that what Western medicine would call an endocrine dysfunction or imbalance cannot be treated by Chinese medicine. It can. However, the way Chinese medicine describes such hormonal dysfunction is very different. All Western hormonal or endocrine functions are all subsumed under the various functions of the Organs, Bowels, and Meridians of traditional Chinese physiology. This is just a different map of the same terrain.

One may ask why classical Chinese doctors did not recognize the endocrine system and its complex, hormonal, metabolic control mechanisms. There are, it seems to me, two reasons for this. First, Chinese medical theory is derived from a cosmological, energetic field theory of how things work in nature which is qualitative, not quantitative. Chinese medicine is based upon the discernment of energetic and functional change, as opposed to chemical and histological change. It is based upon relationships, both within and outside the body, and it tends to look always at the whole picture of the human being within nature, as opposed to any attempt to define smaller and

34

smaller chemical agents (such as hormones) within the body. Western medicine, with its emphasis upon isolation of cellular and molecular structures in the body and specific analysis of chemical components is opposite in its approach.

Secondly, the Chinese doctor of antiquity had no microscope, at least not until this century, and no lab tests are involved in the traditional Chinese diagnostic process. The Chinese medical system of diagnosis is based upon what is referred to as the Four Methods. These include observation with the eyes, auscultation/olfaction or listening/ smelling, questioning of the patient in very specific ways, and palpation, which may consist of feeling the pulse at the radial artery, the courses of the Meridians, and/or the abdominal area. From these Four Methods, the skilled practitioner of TCM can diagnose the condition of all the Organs, tissues, and Meridians of Chinese medicine. What Western science describes as various hormonal or endocrine functions, are categorized in Chinese medicine as functions of these tissues, Organs, or Meridians. Since hormonal imbalance causes changes which can be noted by these four methods of diagnosis, the practitioner of TCM is able to describe a logical disease mechanism for them within the terminology of Chinese medicine. Such Chinese descriptions do allow for effective treatment without knowledge of the specific chemical substances, or hormones involved.

A common problem that the practitioner of Chinese medicine faces with Western clients is the frequent question, "But don't

I REALLY have a hormone imbalance? Can Chinese medicine treat my hormone imbalance?" This question belies a fundamental belief in the ultimate reality of Western science and the answer to this question is both yes and no. Technically speaking, no, the practitioner of Chinese medicine or TCM is treating a Chinese diagnosis which does not talk about hormones or endocrine glands. However, with correct Chinese medical treatment, a Western diagnosis of a hormone imbalance can be effectively treated. Therefore, the answer is also yes, although, technically speaking, a good practitioner of Chinese medicine cannot say so.

## THE MECHANISM OF MENSTRUATION

There are many books available which discuss the hormonal timetable of the menstrual cycle from a Western medical point of view, so that information will not be included here. Chinese medicine has its own theory of the mechanism of menstruation which must be understood if we are also to understand menopause from the Chinese medical perspective.

In Chinese medicine, one name for menstruation is *Tian Kui*, or Heavenly Water. Although this term has many interpretations, for the purposes of this discussion of menopause it is identical to menstruation. As stated above, the arrival of *Tian Kui* is dependent upon a superabundance of Blood which brims over every 28 days or so in the healthy adult female.

36

The creation of Blood is the combined work of three Organs, the Spleen, Heart, and Kidneys. The Spleen distills the essence of digested food and liquids which it sends to the Heart. At the same time, the Kidneys provide a small amount of *Jing* (Vital Essence) which is also sent up to the Heart. Remember from the previous sections that *Jing* is the most primal, essential, fundamental of all substances in the body and is therefore required as a substrate in all metabolic processes resulting in the creation of a pure substance such as Blood. As stated in the Chinese medical classics, the Blood is "turned red" in the Heart. This means that the final transformation of it occurs in the Heart and that the Heart then pumps the Blood out to nourish the rest of the body.

In order for menstruation to occur there must be a surplus of Blood over and above what is required for survival of the body. Prior to puberty, the Organs, in this case especially the Spleen and Kidneys, are not mature. Consequently the production of Qi and Blood is also not mature. Therefore, there is not the surplus or Excess of Blood required for menstruation.

Upon reaching puberty the Spleen and Kidneys are mature. A superabundance of Blood is produced which is stored in the Uterus or Blood Chamber. At this point the Uterus is ready for pregnancy. When sufficient Blood collects there, and if no pregnancy occurs, this Blood brims over, and flows out as the menstruate. The menarche, and the onset of every menstrual period thereafter is called the arrival of *Tian Kui* or Heavenly Water.

At this point we must reiterate that up until recent years practitioners of Chinese medicine had no microscopes and no laboratory tests. They did not know about eggs and sperm, estrogen, progesterone, or other hormones. Understanding of the body, while in many ways quite sophisticated, and in all ways quite logical, was based only upon what the doctor could ascertain through the use of the external senses correlated with an understanding of the functions of the Organs and the flow of the energy and Blood through the Channels and Collaterals.

The Uterus is given many names in the Chinese literature, among them the Fetal Palace, the Fetal Wrapper, the Blood Chamber, and the Wrapper Organ. It is a repository - a storage area, and it is considered one the Six Extraordinary Bowels.[15] The Uterus has relationships with a number of Organs and Meridians which play a part in menstruation and must briefly be described.

The physiological function of the Uterus is first dependent upon the Kidney and the Heart, to which Organs it is connected by two collaterals, or secondary meridians, respectively called the *Bao Luo* and the *Bao Mai*.[16] This implies that menstruation is normal when the Heart (Blood) and Kidney (Qi and *Jing*) are healthy and in proper communication with the Uterus.

38

Additionally, the Spleen plays a role here in that if the Spleen is for any reason weak or compromised, there may not be abundant Blood created from the digestate and first sent up to the Heart to allow for normal menstruation.

Finally, we come the Liver, which plays a major role in the menstrual cycle, having a close relationship with the Uterus. In fact, the Liver is so important to healthy gynecological function that in some literature it is considered the Prenatal Organ in women, as the Kidneys are in men. This is because, as stated above, Blood is the outward physical manifestation of *Jing* in women, and although the Uterus is the Chamber of Blood, it is the Liver which stores the Blood. That is to say, the Liver is responsible for the volume, flow, and regularity of the menstural cycle and for the Blood's nourishing of the tendons and other body tissues as well.

The Liver has another function which relates to menstruation as well. It is responsible for  what is called the patency of Qi flow throughout the body and especially in the pelvis. Patency means smoothness, regularity, and uninterrupted free flow. Since the Qi commands the Blood, these two functions of the Liver are closely related. If the Qi flows unobstructedly, the movement of the Blood will also be regular which means that menstruation will also be normal, on time, and pain free. And, if the Liver stores the Blood properly, the menstrual flow will be normal in volume. Anything which disrupts either of these two functions of the Liver - storage of the Blood and free flow of the Qi - is likely to disrupt menstruation, and will also have a negative impact upon menopause.

Along with the Organs, there are several Meridians which flow through, around, or to the Uterus, and may affect its proper functioning. In addition to the *Bao Luo* and the *Bao Mai* mentioned above, the Kidney, Spleen and Liver meridians all flow through the pelvis with the Liver meridian directly circulating the genitalia. Even more important are two of the so-called Extraordinary meridians, which circulate the pelvis and have an intimate relationship with all female reproductive function. These are the *Ren Mai*, sometimes called the Conception Vessel, and the *Chong Mai*, sometimes called the Penetrating Vessel. The *Ren Mai* circulates mostly Qi in the area of the anterior midline. Its name, Conception Vessel, indicates its close relationship to the Uterus. The *Chong Mai* carries mostly Blood and circulates the central core of the body. It is sometimes said that the the Qi of the *Ren Mai* commands the Blood of the *Chong Mai* and that together these two meridians are largely responsible for the proper female reproductive function. The *Chong Mai* can also be called the Sea of Blood, so one can understand its close connection with the Uterus and Liver. If any of these meridians is blocked, congested, or deficient, there will be consequences in relationship to menstruation and to menopause.

Now that we have introduced all the players, let us discuss the menstrual cycle itself. A normal menstrual cycle should take

28 days, which is roughly divided into four energetic segments of seven days each. Starting with the onset of the period as day one, during the first week the Qi mobilizes the Blood in the Uterus which is full to overflowing at that point. This Blood is moved down and out by the Qi.

During the week after the period, the Blood is relatively Deficient. It takes Blood to enfold and keep the Qi down in the body. If the Blood is insufficient, the Qi, being Yang in nature, will rise like a hot air balloon from which the ballast (Blood) has been ejected. Therefore, the Qi rises toward the upper part of the body.

By midcycle or week three, the Blood has built back up in volume and is no longer Deficient. It begins to accumulate in the Uterus. The Qi has reached its peak in the upper part of the body and begins to be magnetized by the Blood in the pelvis back down into the lower half of the body. This downward movement of the Qi further mobilizes downward even more Blood which accumulates in the Uterus. See Figures 3 and 4.

By week four, the premenstruum, the Qi is trying to descend into the lower half of the body in order to move the Blood down and out. At the same time the Blood is full to Excess, which does not leave much room for the Qi to move freely. It is typically during this week that women with PMS experience physical and emotional symptoms. PMS is often related

41

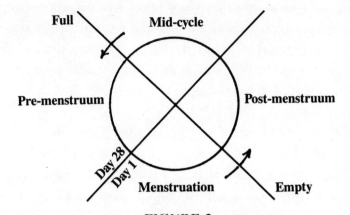

**FIGURE 3.**

**Blood During The Four Phases**
**Of The Menstrual Cycle**

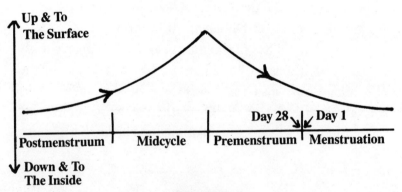

**FIGURE 4.**

**Qi During The Four Phases**
**Of The Menstrual Cycle**

to what is called Liver Qi Stagnation in Chinese medicine. This concept will be discussed in more detail in the next Chapter. If a woman has Liver Qi Stagnation it will tend to manifest by

42

blocking the free flow of energy in the pelvis especially at this time during the menstrual cycle. This Qi Stagnation may be complicated by the fact that if a woman doesn't create enough Blood to magnetize sufficient Qi to the Uterus, the Qi may then flush up to the upper part of the body causing premenstrual headaches, insomnia, breast distention, and other upper body premenstrual signs and symptoms.

When the timetable of menstruation becomes skewed during the menopausal years, any Qi Stagnation will complicate the delicate balancing act that a woman's body is doing, contributing to many of the problems which are loosely grouped together as the menopausal syndrome.

## SUMMARY

This chapter has introduced many of the basic concepts of Traditional Chinese Medicine: Yin/Yang theory, the vital substances, the Organs, meridians, and emotions, and the Chinese medical view of menstruation. While certainly not an exhaustive explication of Chinese medical theory, the information provided here should allow the reader an entrance into the world of Chinese medicine, and should make later chapters describing menopausal disorders understandable. If you have trouble understanding information in later chapters, I suggest that you return to this chapter again for clarification.

# CHAPTER FOUR
# MENOPAUSAL SYNDROME: SIGNS AND SYMPTOMS

Menopause is a naturally occurring transition. *As a physiological event it is not a disease, and it need not be accompanied by any discomfort.* Indeed, statistics show that in 20% of all American women there are no symptoms at all, and in cultures where age brings power and status to women, close to 100% of menopausal women have no reported symptoms.[17]

However, in Western societies where older women are less valued and respected than their younger sisters, approximately 80% of women do have symptoms, ranging from mild and quite transient to severe and debilitating. In Chinese menopausal symptoms are called *Jing Duan Qian Hou Zhu Zheng* or various diseases arising before or after the cessation of menstruation.

In this chapter we will discuss each of the major symptoms associated with menopause, giving the Chinese medical description of the causation or disease mechanism for each one. Treatments and prevention will be dealt with in later chapters.

## THE GENERAL PICTURE

In the *Nei Jing*, the first classic of Chinese medicine, it says that at 14 years of age the Kidneys are mature, the *Chong Mai* becomes full and the *Tian Kui* arrives. A girl reaches puberty and menarche; menstruation begins. This is based on to a Chinese medical theory which describes the physiological growth, maturation, and decline of reproductive function in women in terms of seven year cycles. Each seven year segment describes a state in the natural history of an individual's function, the foundational Organ of Chinese medical physiology. It is said that at seven times seven years (i.e. at 49 years of age) the Kidney Qi begins to decline, the *Tian Kui* is exhausted, and thus the *Chong* and *Ren* meridians are not nourished and menstruation ceases.

Since the *Tian Kui* or menses is the outward manifestation of the *Jing* and of the relationship between the Kidney Qi and the Sea of Blood, a weakening of the Kidney Qi, the *Jing*, and the *Chong Mai* (Sea of Blood) will cause the *Tian Kui* or menstruation to cease. Also, we mentioned that the digestive function begins to decline between 35 and 40 years of age. The net result of this is that less Blood is being created. There is not enough Blood produced every 28 days to create can excess which spills over or is discharged as the menses. These two processes of decline cause the menses to become irregular, the intervals and quantity of Blood become erratic and eventually stop altogether.

In Chapter Three on basic Chinese medical theory it was stated that Yin and Yang must remain in dynamic balance and that Blood and Qi are a Yin Yang pair - the Qi moves the Blood and the Blood is the Mother (substrate or root) of the Qi. Therefore, as less Blood and Body Fluids (Yin) are produced through digestive function, the dynamic balance of Qi to Blood and Yin to Yang begins to come out of balance, with Qi and Yang becoming Excess in relationship to Blood and

Yin. This imbalance compounded by each person's constitutional weaknesses is responsible for most of the problems and disease associated with aging. Furthermore, when this process of decline is accompanied by stress, overwork, emotional upsetment, or any Organic dysfunction in the body, this disequilibrium between Yin and Yang is typically worsened.

This disequilibrium often manifests first as Kidney Yin Deficiency symptoms. However, since Yang requires Yin as its root, a Deficiency of Kidney Yin also eventually leads to a Deficiency of Kidney Yang. As the Kidneys are the root of all Yin and Yang in the body, a Deficiency in the Kidneys may give rise to Deficiency in other Organs. Any Organ may be affected, although different constitutional types tend to manifest the imbalance in different but fairly predictable ways. It is from this general picture that the specific symptoms which we label as part of menopausal syndrome arise. There is, however, one more important concept which we must discuss before we proceed to describe the mechanism for each specific symptom.

# MENOPAUSE, STRESS, AND STAGNATION

With all the possibilities for problems that the simple facts of aging may lead to, why is it that some women experience few or no symptoms and other suffer severe discomfort? Sometimes the reason is purely genetics. Some of us have a stronger constitution, better digestion, or stronger kidneys. Another reason is lifestyle, or how well we have taken care of ourselves over the years. Women who take recreational drugs, drink to excess, smoke, eat poorly, and don't exercise can expect a more difficult menopause than their more health conscious sisters. Sociocultural reasons for menopausal syndrome also exist. How the culture in which a woman finds herself views loss of youth and fertility and, more importantly, how a woman views her life purpose in spite of her cultural milieu can greatly affect whether or not she is symptomatic during her menopause.

According to Chinese medicine, unhealthy lifestyle choices as well as sociocultural stressors all contribute to one basic thing that can make the difference between symptoms and no symptoms during menopause, that being Stagnation. Stagnation is a concept in Chinese medicine which describes any substance or energy in the body which is not flowing or being transformed properly, and hence getting stuck. Six things can become Stagnant in the body according to TCM: Qi, Blood, Food, Dampness, Phlegm, or Fire. (For a more complete

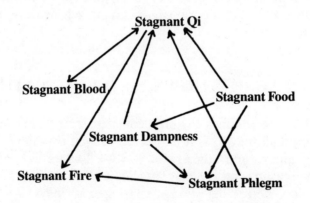

**FIGURE 6.**
Interrelationships of the Six Stagnations

48

discussion of Stagnation in the body, see my previous book, *The Breast Connection: A Laywoman's Guide to The Treatment of Breast Disease by Chinese Medicine,* listed in the Suggested Reading section.) Not only will these Stagnant energies and substances cause different types of problems in the body, but they can and usually do interpromote, with one type of Stagnation leading to or exacerbating another. (See Figure 6). In the case of menopausal problems, however, the most important of all of these is Qi. This is so because of all the Organs, Stagnant Qi most strongly affects the Liver and will worsen any problem related to the Liver. Since the Liver is so strongly connected to the Uterus, the *Chong* and *Ren* Meridians, and the menstrual cycle, any Liver disharmony caused by Stagnant Qi will have a strong impact upon menopause. When Liver Qi Stagnation is combined with the normal decline of Organ function associated with the simple fact of being 45 or 50 years old, the process of menopause is not likely to proceed symptom-free. In most American women, Liver Qi or general Qi Stagnation symptoms will have been present for some time before menopause even begins in the form of digestive difficulties, PMS, breast disease, or frustration and depression.

The most common reason for Stagnant (Liver) Qi is a disturbance of what are called in Chinese medicine the Seven Emotions or the Seven Passions. Another way of stating this is that stress, anger, worry, fear, frustration, boredom, or any other negative emotional state for which a woman has no solution, no outlet, nor the ability to change will cause the Qi to Stagnate. Since we live in a culture that is mostly unsupportive of older women and where we may find our options growing more limited as we get older, certainly it is no wonder that many women are plagued by such feelings. Add to this the generally high level of stress in our culture for women of all ages and the prevalence of Qi Stagnation symptoms this engenders such as irritability and depression, erratic body pains that come and go, fibrocystic breast disease, chronic digestive disorders, and certain aspects of menopausal syndrome become easy to understand.

In the previous chapter I said that the emotions are the subjective mental experience of various manifestations of Qi flow as they relate to various Organs. What is important about this idea is that Qi and the Mind or emotions are not separate, and what happens to one will happen to the other. If some aspect of our lives continually makes us feel stuck, dissatisfied, or limited, then over time that is what will happen to our Qi as well. This means that our mental/emotional state is most important in either producing or preventing Qi Stagnation symptoms. We will discuss this point more in the sections on self-help treatment.

Stagnation of Qi can cause problems enough by itself - distention and bloating, cramping pain, emotional lability. But as stated above, it will usually lead to other types of problems, complicate problems that already exist, or destabilize any delicate energetic transition that the body is going through, such as menopause. This is because if not remedied, Stagnant Qi will transform into pathogenic Heat.

Warmth is an inherent quality of Qi and of life itself, so that if enough of it Stagnates in one place for a long enough period of time, it will become hot, or transform to (Stagnant) Fire. Excessive Heat such as this has a number of effects. It dries out the Blood and Yin of the body which, in menopausal women, are already compromised by the fact of aging. This leads to further imbalance of Qi to Blood and Yin to Yang. Further, since Blood and Yin are required to root or anchor Qi and Yang, if this imbalance becomes too great, the Qi/Yang

50

will rise up and to the Surface of the body like a hot air balloon. This is how hot flashes, night sweats, headaches, irritability, dry eyes, and certain types of vertigo and insomnia arise.

Another scenario that can happen when Stagnant Qi becomes Stagnant Fire is that the Blood can become overheated. The Qi commands the Blood and is responsible for its movement, so that if the Qi is Hot it may transfer this Heat to the Blood. Just like water boiling over on the stove, the Blood will "boil over" and run recklessly outside its Channels. This causes erratic or excessive bleeding during the period or at unscheduled times between periods. This condition may be further exacerbated by Qi Deficiency. If Qi and Blood are Stagnated, then fresh Qi and Blood cannot be created efficiently. Since another inherent function of the Qi is to restrain the Blood and hold it within its Channels, if the Qi is insufficient for this job, the Blood will not be held in and further bleeding can happen. Bleeding due to Excessive Heat in the Blood and Qi Deficiency is typically large in volume, whereas bleeding caused by low grade Heat is more often scant. Both of these are common problems during menopause.

In addition to problems with bleeding, long term Stagnant Liver Qi can also become what is called Depressive Liver Fire which can lead to painful breasts, a stuffy, oppressed sensation in the chest, a bitter taste in the mouth, irritability and irascibility alternating with bouts of depression, and possibly bleeding gums, headaches, or toothaches if this Fire vents up.

A third possible way in which Qi Stagnation can aggravate the menopausal situation is if there is already a tendency to Kidney Yang/Spleen Yang Deficiency. According to the Chinese medical theory of Five Elements or Five Phases, Liver Wood

51

must control Spleen (Earth) just a tree prevents erosion of the soil. If the Spleen is already weak, then the Liver may overexert this control on the Spleen, making it even weaker. The Spleen is the Organ which, when weak, is responsible for the production of Pathogenic Phlegm and Dampness. If the Spleen is made weaker by overcontrol or invasion from a Stagnant and overheated Liver, there will tend to be even more Phlegm and Dampness, leading to edema, loose stools, obesity, and more seriously, lumps and bumps in the flesh or in the Organs. Furthermore, if the Liver is overheated, these lumps and bumps can become solidified, like gooey dumplings which harden into bread when steamed or boiled. This is one way that tumors, both benign and

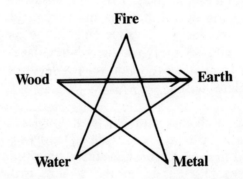

**FIGURE 7.**
**Liver Wood Invades Spleen Earth**

malignant, are created. What's worse, if Phlegm and Dampness are present for any length of time, they will exacerbate Stagnant Qi, similarly to how a flooded road impedes the normal flow of traffic. Thus, we again see how various Stagnant factors, in this case Dampness and Qi, may interpromote, each making the other worse. (See Figure 7 above.)

Liver Qi Stagnation will also effect the Lungs adversely. According to Five Phase Theory, each Organ is responsible for the control of one other Organ so that none become Excess or too strong.(See Figure 8.) It is the Lung's job to control the Liver. When the Liver becomes congested or Stagnant, this is a species of Excess. If the Liver gets too powerful, it will turn around and attack the Lungs which are supposed to keep it in check. (See Figure 9.) In such cases there may be chronic cough, but even if there is no cough, weak Lungs can contribute to hot flashes and night sweats, the mechanism for which is described in more detail under hot flashes below.

Finally, Liver Qi Stagnation can aggravate the Heart. Because the relationship of Qi and Blood is a Yin Yang relationship, if the Qi (Yang) becomes Stagnant and Hot, the Blood (Yin) will become evaporated and exhausted. Exhausted Blood primarily affects the Liver and the Heart. The Liver and Heart respectively are responsible for "housing" or "treasuring" the *Hun*, (Psyche, Ego) and the *Shen* (Spirit, Mind). It is the Blood in the Liver and Heart which is responsible for doing this job. Therefore, if the Liver Blood and Heart Blood have been exhausted by Heat, the Spirit will be unable to "rest" or remain calm in the Heart and the Psyche/Ego will be unable to remain calm in the Liver. This leads to such symptoms as palpitations, insomnia, restlessness, anxiety, poor memory, emotional lability, and dream-disturbed sleep.

53

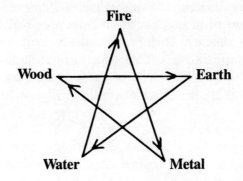

**FIGURE 8.**
**Control *(Ke)* Cycle Of Five Phase Theory**

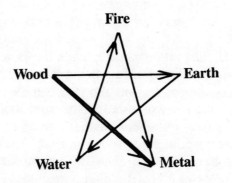

**FIGURE 9.**
**Liver Insults the Lung**

While many of these symptoms may arise without the aggravation of Liver Qi Stagnation, its presence will most assuredly

54

aggravate any tendency that a woman may have toward these symptoms, and its absence may spell the difference between health and the lack of it during the menopause. It is rather like the proverbial straw on the camel's back. The good news is that, unlike the normal decline in Qi, Blood, Yin, and *Jing* which accompanies and is identical to aging, Liver Qi Stagnation can be controlled, if not completely eradicated.

With all this information about Qi Stagnation in mind, let us go on to the details of some of the specific symptoms of menopausal syndrome.

## HOT FLASHES

This is by far the most common symptom women experience during menopause. According to Chinese medicine it is caused by Deficiency of Kidney Yin of the Kidneys and Liver, and the consequent rising of Liver Yang to the upper part of the body. Earlier we spoke of Yin being related to water, moistening, coolness, and structure, and Yang being related to fire, brightness, and to upward, swift, hot movement. A hot flash is a Yang event in the body, the swift upward movement of Heat to the Surface and especially the chest and head. But this swift erratic movement of Heat is due to an underlying Deficiency of its opposite, Water or Yin. Yin is required to enfold, control, root and lower, the Yang of the body. If Kidney Yin is insufficient, the Yang energy has no Root to hold it down, no ballast to keep it from rising, and it therefore floats up out of control to the upper part of the body.

Typically, the Lungs are also involved in hot flashes. The Lungs control the *Wei* Qi or Hot Defensive energy produced by Kidney Yang in the pelvis. This control is exerted by the Lungs' commanding the opening and closing of the pores.

55

Since most women with menopausal complaints also suffer from Liver Qi and since Excess Liver Qi insults and weakens the Lungs according to classical Five Phase theory, often the Lungs are too weak to adequately astringe the Surface and keep the pores shut. See Fig.9. This is especially the case when hot flashes are accompanied by sweating. Since sweat is the Fluid of the Heart, such abnormal and recurrent sweating exhausts Heart Yin and Blood and further leads to anxiousness, mental instability, and palpitations. This is because the Heart *Shen* or Spirit is nurtured and rooted in Heart Yin and Blood. Since the Heart and Lungs are the two Organs that descend especially Qi and Fluids and Blood, weakening of these two Organs exacerbates any tendency for flushing up.

## NIGHT SWEATS

The mechanism for night sweats is exactly the same as for hot flashes but with a slight twist. The Surface Qi of the body, called *Wei* or Defensive Qi, is the most Yang aspect of the Qi. It moves quickly, is aggressive, and controls perspiration. During the day it stays on the Surface of the body. At night it is withdrawn into the core of the body to warm and protect the Organs. Whether due either to a normal or pathological reason, when this Qi moves rapidly out to the Surface of the body with rising Heat, the Body Fluids in the skin (perspiration) move out with it. Perspiration, according to Chinese medicine, is a Pure Fluid. It is not a discharge of something foul, fetid, or unnecessary. While normal perspiration with exertion or in hot weather is normal, its excessive, uncontrolled, or untimely loss is not considered healthy. Especially when the body is at rest and not exerting itself, no sweat should appear. Night sweating is a classic symptom of what is called Yin Deficiency Heat or Fire.

56

Since Yin rules or relates to the night hours and the darkness, if the Yin is weak, symptoms of its weakness are all the more prevalent during that time. It is during the night especially that Yin must do its job of overpowering and enfolding the Yang, including the *Wei* Qi. If Yin is Deficient, it cannot hold and enfold the Yang and the *Wei* Qi or *Wei* Yang flushes to the Surface bringing with it again Body Fluids in the form of sweat. This is because it is the Yang Qi which mobilizes and transports fluids. When Yin and Yang are in relative balance[18] night sweating does not occur.

## INSOMNIA

Some women say that the insomnia they have during meno-pause is due to the night sweats which awaken them, drenched and flushed, having to change their night clothes. Chinese medicine does not necessarily say that it is the night sweats which cause the interruption of sleep so much as that they occur concommitently.

In the previous chapter we spoke about each of the five major Organs being responsible for, or related to, one of the Five Spirits or aspects of the psychoemotional make-up. Sleep problems are mostly related to the Heart, which "houses" the *Shen* (Mind or Spirit), and/or the Liver, which "houses" the *Hun* (Psyche or Ego). This relationship was mentioned above in the discussion of Qi Stagnation and its potential ramifications with various Organs. The *Shen* and the *Hun* together comprise consciousness. Compared to Blood and Yin which nourish and root them, they are both Yang. If the *Shen* and *Hun* cannot be housed properly, sleep will not be calm. The ability of the Heart and Liver to do this job is directly related to a healthy supply of Blood and Yin. Systemic Blood Defi-ciency due to a decline of Spleen and/or Kidney function will

57

most often affect the Heart or the Liver, often resulting in insomnia or dream-disturbed sleep. This again can be seen as the Yang energy flushing up due to Yin energy being insufficient to enfold and hold it.

Systemic Blood Deficiency is a common problem in menopausal women. The cessation of the period is, as stated earlier, a sign of the body's declining ability to create Blood. It is, therefore, not unreasonable to think that some women might experience symptoms of Blood Deficiency, insomnia being among them.

Additionally, the Blood is a part of the Yin of the body and Yin is responsible for rest and sleep. If the Root of Yin, the Kidney Yin, is Deficient, which as we have seen is a common situation in menopausal women, sleep disturbance is a typical consequence of this decline. If there is, as it so often is in American women, the complication of Liver Qi Stagnation, the Spleen will also typically be Deficient, thus reducing Blood production to nurture the Heart and Liver. Furthermore, Liver Qi Stagnation, which is a form of local Excess, almost always implies Liver Blood Deficiency. Qi and Blood form a dynamic Yin Yang relationship and it is a basic premise of Yin Yang theory that when Yang flourishes, Yin in consumed[19].

To summarize all this, weakening of Yin leads to a preponderance of Yang and Yang is consciousness or wakefulness. Insufficiency of Blood prevents the Spirit from resting calmly in the Heart, and/or the Psyche from resting in the Liver. This is the basic scenario of insomnia in menopausal women.

## IRRITABILITY AND DEPRESSION

These two emotional problems, so common in Western

58

menopausal women, are like two sides of the same coin, and in some women will alternate back and forth, or even occur together. These emotional symptoms are largely due to Liver Qi Stagnation, usually over a long period of time.

First the Liver Qi becomes Excess, loses its patency and cannot flow smoothly. If this situation is unresolved, this stuck Qi transforms to Heat. If this Heat remains stuck and congested and is unable to move or change, depression will occur. If the Heat comes unstuck and rises in fits and starts, this will often manifest as bursts or fits of anger and irritability which may be inappropriate to the situation. Anger and irritability are Hot emotions. These two situations may alternate, or one may be predominant depending upon the case.

Unfortunately, if the Liver remains congested and Hot, the Blood and Yin will be further dried out and damaged. This exacerbates the imbalance that already exists creating a vicious cycle. This is one reason that depression is such a difficult symptom to treat effectively. In fact, in cases of severe clinical depression, that Western drug therapy is often necessary while trying to deal with the root of the problem with more natural methods.

**NERVOUSNESS AND ANXIETY**

Nervousness and anxiety, like insomnia, are related to the Heart. As was stated before, the Heart must be replete with Blood in order for the Spirit to rest calmly. When Heart Blood is Deficient, the Spirit has no home or resting place. It therefore flits about like a restless bird, unable to land for long in one place. Our subjective experience of this is a nervous, restless, anxious mental state which may improve or get worse depending upon the level of systemic or Heart Blood Deficiency which is, in turn, related to diet, work, stress, and even how much love is in our life. One highly respected Chinese medical practitioner once told me that one cannot make Blood when the Heart is longing. Since sufficient Blood is such an important factor in women's health this supports the hypothesis that psychoemotional and social factors play an important role in determining a woman's overall health at any time in life.

## FATIGUE

Fatigue, according the Chinese medicine, is always related to Qi Deficiency. Movement, activity, and energy to do anything are Yang by Chinese definition. Since Qi is the aspect of Yang which is responsible for motion, action, aliveness, or pep, a shortage of Qi will lead to the opposite condition -- lethargy, fatigue, and exhaustion. However, once again we must remember the Yin/Yang relationship of Qi to Blood. Since Blood is the mother of the Qi, Blood deficiency can also lead to Qi Deficiency, or exacerbate any tendency to Qi Deficiency. Therefore, fatigue is also often associated with Blood Deficiency as well.

The Organs most involved in fatigue are the Spleen, Lungs, and Kidneys. The Spleen's job is to transform Qi and Blood from the essence of digested food and liquids. The Lungs' job is to circulate the Qi to the body Surface and to send it down to the Kidneys. The Kidneys' job is to grasp the Qi which the Lungs descend, energizing the lower body, and to provide the basic Fire of Life which is the pilot light for the Stomach/Spleen. The process of creating energy from what we ingest and what we breathe is a process of burning, cooking, or combustion. As has been mentioned several times, the digestive fire of the Stomach/Spleen begins to weaken at some point in our late 30's or early 40's. Parenthetically, this is why we often put on weight at about that time even though our diet and activity remain the same.

If our diet is not a healthy one or if it requires more fire than what is available in the Stomach/Spleen, two things can happen. First the Kidneys will be required to work harder to provide more Heat/Qi to assist the Stomach/Spleen with the logical possibility of them also becoming depleted. If the Kidneys cannot make up this deficit or become weak trying to do so, then there will be signs of both Spleen Qi Deficiency and Kidney Qi Deficiency. Since the function that we are talking about here has to do with Heat, it will be the Yang aspect of the Kidneys and Spleen that is most likely to be affected. Initially the symptoms may include fatigue, listlessness, fluctuations in appetite, chronic mild diarrhea, or other digestive disturbances. More serious Qi Deficiency may manifest as anemia, dysfunctional uterine bleeding, prolapse of the stomach, uterus, rectum, or bladder, cold limbs, frequent watery diarrhea, a tendency to easy bruising, nausea, heaviness of the chest or head, or chronic gastroenteritis. These are all Spleen Qi and Yang Deficiency signs and symptoms. If the Kidneys also become Deficient trying to help out the Spleen, further symptoms may include low back pain, sciatica, lack of will power, loss of sex drive, frequent urination, or urinary incontinence. These are typical Kidney Deficiency signs and symptoms.

Fatigue, therefore, is an initial sign of Qi Deficiency usually starting with the Spleen. This is one reason why a good diet is so important during menopause and all the time really. An entire section will be devoted to diet in Chapter Eight on prevention and self-help.

61

## PALPITATIONS

Palpitations are another Heart symptom. However, they can be caused by a number of disease mechanisms. In most menopausal syndrome cases they are due to Heart Blood Deficiency, Heart Yin Deficiency, or Heart Fire Flaring. These may all be aggravated or complicated by flaring upward of Liver/Stomach Heat

Heart Blood Deficiency we have discussed above in relationship to the Spleen. At menopause it is weaker and not supplying the Heart with enough raw materials to transform Blood properly. Without sufficient Blood, the Heart Qi lacks its foundation, and the function, i.e. the heartbeat, becomes irregular. Since Qi moves the Blood, if Heart Qi becomes weak, it may not be sufficient to keep the Blood flowing and so there are interruptions in the beat.

The source of Heart Yin Deficiency is not related to the Spleen but to the Kidneys, and to some extent the Lungs. In several places above the Kidneys have been mentioned as the source of True Yin or Original Yin. A Deficiency of any aspect of Kidney energy will almost always affect other Organs as well. Also, we have said that the Heart and Kidney are connected via the internal channels called the *Bao Luo* and *Bao Mai* and also via the *Chong Mai*. Many or even most menopausal symptoms are related to Kidney Yin Deficiency. If the Kidney Yin is Deficient then the Yin of the Liver, Heart, and Lungs also tends to become Deficient. Said more simply, Kidney Yin Deficiency often leads to Heart, Liver and, Lung Yin Deficiency via several internal channels. In the case of the Heart, when Kidney Yin is Deficient the Kidney and Liver Yang will rise, and overheat the Heart. When overheated, the Heart Qi will move too fast and the Heart Blood will become dried out from this Heat. The exhausted Blood will no longer be able to hold onto the Qi and function as its substrate. This coming apart of the Qi and Blood is experienced as a palpitation. The Qi comes apart from the Blood which it is moving and skips ahead like a stone skipping over water.

Another possible scenario for menopausal palpitations is Heat flushing up from the Liver and Stomach into the upper body. Heat in the Liver is typically due to Kidney Yin being Deficient and not keeping the Liver moist and cool, Liver Qi Stagnation transforming to Heat, excessive consumption of greasy, spicy foods, or some combination of these factors. Although the Stomach can become Hot without Liver the two typically become Hot together because of their close relationship. As stated before, when enough Heat collects in one place it rises. If Heat from the Liver and Stomach flush upward both the Heart and Lungs can be affected. Another attribute of Heat is that it will speed up the movement of Qi. In this case the Heart Qi speeds up and comes apart from the Blood which has been dried out or damaged by the Heat as well. This is experienced as a palpitation.

These etiologies for palpitations are related may combine and interpromote in some women. Again we see the importance of a healthy diet and the control of stress factors which lead to Liver Qi Stagnation.

## NAUSEA/DIARRHEA/CONSTIPATION

These are mostly due to a disharmony between the Liver and Spleen/Stomach. Liver Wood must control the unchecked growth of Spleen/Stomach Earth. When the Liver becomes congested or Excess it is common for Wood to invade Earth. When this happens, the Spleen typically becomes Deficient and

Damp. Whereas, the Stomach becomes Hot and Excess along with the Liver. Spleen Damp and Deficiency leads to loss of appetite, fatigue, and diarrhea. Stomach Excess causes nausea, belching and Heartburn. Diarrhea can also be aggravated by any tendency to Kidney Yang Deficiency.

The typical cause of menopausal constipation is somewhat different. Earlier it was stated that one of the Liver's jobs is to move the Qi in a smooth, patent, free-flowing manner. This includes the Large Intestine Qi. When the Liver Qi is congested, it loses its ability to maintain this fee flow, often resulting in poor Large Intestine motility and peristalsis. Add to this a general drying of the Yin or moisture in the body and the bowels then are not only difficult to move, but the stools themselves may become dry, hard, and difficult to pass. In TCM terminology, such constipation is described as being due to a combination of Liver Qi Stagnation and Fluid Dryness of the Large Intestine.

In addition to the Qi Stagnation and Fluid Dryness, weakness of Kidney Yang may also play a role in causing constipation in menopausal and postmenopausal women. The functions of Kidney Yang energy include controlling the process that transforms and circulates water through the body. When Kidney Yang is Deficient, as is common in older people, the process of warming and transforming water is weakened. Too much water is excreted by the Bladder resulting in clear and copious urination. This disruption in the proper circulation of water in the pelvis dries out the Intestines complicating the above mechanism of constipation.

**STIFFNESS & CRAMPS**

According to Chinese medicine, the tendons and ligaments are nourished by Liver Blood. When exercising it is the Liver which sends out enough Blood to allow the tendons and ligaments strength and flexibility. When Liver Blood becomes Deficient, the tendons and ligaments cannot be nourished properly, leading to cramping, stiffness, and pain. The mechanism for why Liver Blood becomes Deficient at menopause has already been discussed in several prior sections above.

## JOINT PAIN

The joints are nourished and kept limber and smooth by the action of the Yin Fluids of the body. In Chinese medicine, the joints are believed to be ruled by the Kidneys and specifically relate to Kidney Yin. If the True Yin or Kidney Yin becomes Deficient, all the Yin of the body will be affected, including all Body Fluids. When these are Deficient, the joints can become painful and lose their flexibility. Pain in the spinal vertebrae due to bone demineralization is covered below.

## VAGINAL DRYNESS

The vagina is also kept moist, soft, and lubricated by the Body Fluids. Additionally, the genitals are ruled by the Kidney and Liver. If Kidney/Liver Yin is Deficient, the Body Fluids in the genital area will be affected. If there is also Liver Qi Stagnation, the genitals will tend to become dried out due to transformative Heat in the Liver meridian, which directly circulates the genitalia. This not only causes dryness but chronic inflammation and/or itching. Persistent vaginal discomfort may also contribute to loss of interest in sex.

## BONE DEMINERALIZATION / OSTEOPOROSIS

According to TCM, the Kidneys rule the bones, teeth, head

hair, ears, and the marrow of the spinal cord and brain. If symptoms arise in these areas of the body, the Chinese medical practitioner always investigates for Kidney involvement. Since we know the Kidneys are already in a natural state of decline by the time of menopause, the bones will also be declining. Since the substance of any part of the body is the Yin part, loss of bone substance is related to the decline of Kidney Yin. Fortunately, there are many things a woman can do to prevent bone demineralization and avoid osteoporosis. These are discussed in the chapter on prevention and in Appendix II.

## ABNORMAL OR EXCESSIVE BLEEDING

Chinese medical theory describes abnormal bleeding of any type as due to one or a combination of three causes: Heat, Blood Stagnation, or Qi Deficiency. In menopausal women abnormal uterine bleeding is typically due to some combination of at least two of these, and in some cases all three. As described earlier on page 51, long term Qi Stagnation may lead to what is called Depressive Heat causing the Blood to boil over and run recklessly outside its pathways. Addi- tionally, Heat due to Deficient Yin which is so common in menopausal women may worsen any tendency to Depressive Heat. Second- ly, since it is Qi which holds the Blood within its pathways, Deficient Qi may be too weak to perform this func- tion, allowing the Blood to fall or leak out. Finally, Blood Stagna- tion creates blockage causing the Blood to flow outside its normal pathways rather like a traffic jam with cars driving down the shoulders or median strip in order to keep moving.

## LOSS OF SEX DRIVE

This is a very upsetting symptom for most women and may adversely   affect relationships   with husbands or lovers. Vaginal discomfort and dryness may play a role here, but other

Vaginal discomfort and dryness may play a role here, but other disease mechanisms also usually play a part. Sexual desire is a function of Kidney Yang -- the Fire of the Kidneys, sometimes called the *Ming Men Huo*, or Life Gate Fire. Kidney Yang normally declines slowly with age, but most women do not experience this decline in its true form at menopause because Kidney Yin is declining more rapidly at this time. However, when Kidney Yin declines, the Kidney Yang floats up because it has no root leaving the pelvic area relatively deficient of Yang energy. Therefore, a woman feels no desire for sex. Since Yin and Yang are interdependent, if Yin is not reconsolidated fairly quickly, the Yang may also become Deficient, and a true Yang Deficiency will develop, leading to more exaggerated symptoms. If on the other hand a woman's body reorganizes effectively after the menses stops and her Yin is properly rebuilt, the Yang will once again have a root, and normal sexual desire will return.

## EARLY MENOPAUSE AND ARTIFICIAL MENOPAUSE

Although not specifically symptoms of menopause, early menopause and artificial menopause are not uncommon phenomenon in our culture and deserve some discussion. Early menopause is described by Western medicine as menopause which occurs prior to the age of 40, having many potential causes. Having made a diagnosis of early menopause, Western medicine dismisses such women with the prescription of estrogen replacement therapy. According to Chinese medical theory, early menopause indicates that a woman has aged prematurely. That is to say, her biological age has exceeded her chronological age. Usually this indicates decline in Kidney *Jing* or in both Kidney Yin and Liver Blood. Chinese medicine does not consider early menopause to be normal or healthy; it means a woman has aged prematurely

67

beyond her years. Effective treatments for reversing it are available using herbal and orthomolecular therapy. When such treatment is effective, it means that Chinese medicine has succeeded in rolling back the biological age of these women resulting in their being biologically younger.

Surgical menopause, that is menopause due to the removal of the uterus, does not seem to be reversible either by Chinese or Western medicine no matter what the age of the woman. However, if a woman is thrown into artificial menopause by surgery prior to the age of 49, she is still producing a superabundance of Blood which no longer has an avenue for discharge. This Excess Blood may lead to Blood Stagnation which, in turn, may lead to abdominal masses or neoplasms. Appropriate Chinese medical treatment can eliminate or at least mitigate the effects of such Blood Stagnation and it potential consequences in these women.

Radiation and chemotherapy cause artificial menopause because they injure and deplete the *Jing* and Blood. While Chinese medical treatment may not be able to reestablish menstruation in these women, it can help replenish the *Jing* and Blood enough to retard the aging process which the artificial menopause implies.

## OTHER SYMPTOMS

Other symptoms that occasionally appear with menopause may include dizziness, vertigo, headaches, blurring vision, tinnitus, excessive thirst, edema, cold limbs, low back pain, weight gain, poor appetite, and memory loss. These are all related to one or more of the basic diagnostic patterns of disharmony which account, alone or in combination, for menopausal discomfort. These patterns are discriminated in detail in the next chapter.

## CHAPTER FIVE
# THE TCM DIAGNOSIS OF MENOPAUSAL SYNDROME

Diagnosis in TCM is based on the discrimination of professionally recognized, named patterns of disharmony. Traditional
Chinese diagnostic patterns are differentiated based on signs
and symptoms, observation of the tongue, and palpation of the
pulse, abdomen, and Meridians. They are not based on
laboratory tests. Traditional Chinese patterns of disharmony
are usually directly descriptive of the patient's experience of
their dis-ease.

Also, the descriptive patterns used in Chinese medicine are
derived from a direct observation of phenomena in the natural
world. Let us take for example the pattern called Wind. As
a natural phenomenon Wind comes out of nowhere, is fast
moving, comes and goes in fits and starts, and causes things to
move, shake, tremble, or change shape. Wind as a diagnostic
pattern describes exactly the same qualities. Wind diseases
come on rapidly, move quickly, possibly from one part of the
body to another, can come and go unexpectedly, and cause
involuntary movement. Further, because Wind manifests in
Heaven or the sky, Wind diseases also typically manifest in the
upper part of the body.

TCM diagnostic patterns are classified in several ways. The

69

first way patterns may be subdivided is whether they are Meridian patterns, Organ/Bowel patterns, or patterns related to specific tissues in the body. The second subdivision is slightly more complex, dividing patterns by what are called the Eight Principle Patterns: Hot/Cold, Excess/Deficiency, External/Internal, Yin/Yang. Thirdly, patterns are subdivided according to whether they involve the body humors: Qi, Blood, Body Fluids, and *Jing*. Finally, patterns may be classified according to Five Phase or Five Element theory.

In actual practice, these pattern categories are combined when diagnosing a single patient thus giving a great deal of texture and complexity to pattern identification. Each individual pattern has its professionally agreed upon signs and symptoms. However, real life patients almost always suffer from a combination of two or more such patterns of disharmony and so their signs and symptoms are likewise a mixture. Textbooks must describe these patterns as distinct, but few patients present such neatly packaged signs and symptoms. For this reason, TCM practitioners practice for years before really developing the skill to move from such simple textbook discriminations to diagnosing complex real life patients.

Happily, in menopausal syndrome only a few of these patterns predominate. That is because disharmony in women's bodies tends to arise in specific ways at specific times in our lives depending upon our constitutional make-up. In fact, based upon a woman's constitution at 30 or 35, a good practitioner of Chinese medicine should be able to predict quite accurately what type of menopausal problems, if any, a woman is likely to experience and perhaps offer her preventive suggestions.

Below are the major patterns of disharmony which account for most menopausal symptoms, with a description of the signs and symptoms defining each pattern. However, remember that, as just stated, these patterns can, and often do combine with each other or with other patterns related to a woman's constitutional tendencies to make the overall picture of a woman's health more complicated. Rarely will a woman's situation be as simple as one or another of these patterns alone.

## LIVER BLOOD KIDNEY YIN DEFICIENCY

Liver Blood Kidney Yin Deficiency is the main mechanism for the cessation of menstruation. Menses stops because there is insufficient Liver Blood and Kidney Yin of *Jing* to support it. In women where this dual deficiency is more severe, however, it may also result in other signs and symptoms. These include:

-hot flashes/sweating, especially in the upper body
-headaches, blurred vision, dizziness, vertigo, tinnitus, spots in front of the eyes
-weakness/soreness of lower back or legs
-constipation
-thirst or dry mouth
-insomnia or dream-disturbed sleep

Tongue: red, with little or no coating or a dry scant yellow coating
Pulse: thready, wiry, and rapid

These signs and symptoms are due to a drying up of Yin below. This causes Fluid Dryness constipation and weakness or soreness of the low back and legs due to lack of Blood nourishing the sinews and tendons. This also results in Yang energy floating upward due to its lack of root in the Yin below. This results in hot flashes, night sweats, dizziness, blurred vision, insomnia, and a dry mouth. This is the most common

71

menopausal pattern of disharmony. It arises due to an imbalance of Yin and Yang, based upon the decline of the Kidneys and the general tendency for Yang to be Excess in relationship to Yin as we grow older. No matter what other patterns may complicate an individual woman's menopause, the vast majority of women with menopausal complaints have this pattern at the root of these complaints.

## ASCENDANT LIVER YANG

Ascendant Liver Yang is derived from Liver Qi Stagnation which undergoes transformation due to the previous pattern. The pure signs and symptoms of this pattern are:

-dizziness and vertigo
-tinnitus and red eyes
-menopausal migraines
-a bitter taste in the mouth
-irritability and even irascibility
-hot flashes and sweats
-profuse menstrual flow due to Heat in the Blood
-lingering menstrual flow or spotting

Tongue: red
Pulse: wiry and rapid

These signs and symptoms describe more forceful ascension of Yang energy to the upper part of the body than the previous pattern. The previous pattern's signs and symptoms describe Deficiency Heat rising whereas Ascendant Liver Yang symptoms are due to Excess Yang. The mechanism for the signs and symptoms are not different as both have to do with a flushing up of Yang. The difference lies in degree. This technical difference is important when it comes to TCM therapeutics. Often Kidney Yin Liver Blood Deficiency is complicated by Ascension of Liver Yang.

## KIDNEY AND SPLEEN YANG DEFICIENCY

In this pattern, symptoms mostly reflect Cold and Dampness accumulating in the body due to an inability of Spleen and Kidney Yang to transport and transform Body Fluids.

>    -pale complexion
>    -limbs and body cold and an aversion to cold
>    -lower back pain, cold lower back
>    -loss of appetite
>    -clear copious urine or
>    -very scant urine accompanied by edema
>    -abdominal distention
>    -early morning diarrhea or tendency to loose stools
>    -loss of sex drive
>    -obesity

Tongue: pale, swollen with a white or wet coating
Pulse: deep, weak, and/or slow

In a small proportion of menopausal cases, Kidney Yang is weaker than Yin, in which case symptoms related to coldness and poor water metabolism will arise. In Western medicine, this syndrome may present as edema, various digestive disturbances, prolapse of various organs, or functional uterine bleeding.

## ACCUMULATION OF PHLEGM AND STAGNATION OF QI

This pattern is due to the decline of Spleen function in its processing of Liquids. As mentioned above, Liver Qi leads to

Spleen Deficiency and Dampness. Likewise, decline of Kidney Yang also leads to Spleen Deficiency since the root of the Spleen's ability to transform and transport is derived from the heat of the Kidneys. It is said in Chinese medicine that the Spleen is the root of Phlegm production. Phlegm is due to the congelation of Dampness. This is aggravated by any tendency towards Liver Heat which brews the Fluids cooking them into Phlegm. Once Phlegm is created it tends to block the flow of Qi, thus aggravating Liver Qi. It may also obstruct what in Chinese medicine are called the orifices of the Heart. This results in various mental/emotional symptoms. Although this pattern rarely causes menopausal signs and symptoms by itself, it does often complicate and aggravate all the other, more common patterns associated with menopausal complaints. The signs and symptoms of Accumulation of Phlegm and Stagnation of Qi are:

-stuffy chest and chest oppression
-depression
-fear and anxiety
-palpitations
-insomnia
-copious mucous
-a possible lump in the throat
-nausea or vomiting
-obesity

Tongue: darkish with a turbid, greasy coating
Pulse: slippery and wiry

## HEART BLOOD AND SPLEEN QI DEFICIENCY

Spleen Qi catalyzes the creation of Heart Blood. If the Spleen Qi is Deficient, over time Heart Blood will also become

74

Deficient. Constant stress and mental overwork may also lead to this condition. The symptoms of Heart Blood Spleen Qi Deficiency are:

 -palpitations and shortness of breath
 -anxiety or emotional instability
 -loss of memory
 -insomnia and/or excessive dreams
 -pale or yellowish complexion
 -tendency to fatigue
 -itchy skin

Tongue: pale and flabby with teeth indentations on the sides.
Pulse: fine and weak or deficient

## HEART YIN AND BLOOD DEFICIENCY

This pattern is due to the Heart Yin and Blood not being transformed and thus failing to nourish and secure the Heart Spirit. Because Heart Yin is rooted in Kidney Yin, decline of Liver and Kidney Yin may result in Heart Yin Deficiency. And because the Spleen and Liver are the two Organs which participate in the control of Blood, if Spleen Qi no longer transforms Blood and the Liver no longer stores Blood as efficiently as previously, Heart Blood may become Deficient. In addition, since Heart Blood and Yin are both species of Yin they are mutually interdependent.

The signs and symptoms of Heart Yin and Blood Deficiency primarily have to do with the Blood and Yin's failure in nourishing the function of the Heart and the Heart Spirit. This results in:

 -dream-disturbed sleep

75

-palpitations
-loss of memory
-insomnia

If Heart Yin Deficiency predominates,the signs and symptoms will be:

-restlessness
-heat in the palms, soles, and center of the chest
-afternoon low-grade fever
-night sweats
-racing of the heart

Tongue:  If Heart Blood Deficiency predominates the tongue is pale. If Heart Yin Deficiency predominates the tongue is red.
Pulse: If Heart Blood Deficiency is predominant the pulse is fine and forceless.  If Heart Yin Deficiency is predominant the pulse is fine and rapid.

## HEART AND KIDNEYS NOT COMMUNICATING

This pattern describes a situation where, due to loss of capillary attraction and mutual restraint of Fire and Water in the body, a woman experiences Hot symptoms in the upper body and Deficient Yin symptoms in the lower.  Fire blazes up and Water dribbles down. According to Five Phase theory, the Water of the Kidney should maintain communication with and control over the Fire in the Heart.  When this communication is lost the following symptoms will appear.

-insomnia
-nervousness and anxiety
-palpitations

-frequent dreams
-leukorrhea or excessive vaginal discharge
-incontinence or dribbling urination
-uterine bleeding

Tongue: red tip, apically fluted, scant coating
Pulse: fast, floating, or flooding

The difference between this Heat above and Deficient Yin below and that of the previously described patterns is that the signs and symptoms of heat primarily manifest as disruptions in Heart function according to TCM. This pattern therefore, specifically describes a Heart/Kidney imbalance as opposed to a more general Yin Yang disequilibrium.

This pattern differs from the preceding patterns in that there is Deficiency Fire flaring upward in the Heart disturbing the Spirit. Whereas in the preceding pattern the Spirit is simply malnourished.

**DEFICIENCY OF YIN AND YANG OF THE KIDNEY**

This pattern is again a mixture of both Hot and Cold symptoms. It often appears as Hot symptoms above and Cold symptoms below. Since the Yin of the Kidneys is weak, whatever weak Yang there is in the body is not rooted and floats up, leaving the lower body Yang Deficient and therefore Cold. Varying symptoms may arise including:

-cold lower limbs and low back feel cold
-body feels like it is sitting in cold water from the waist
     down
-afternoon flushes of the face, neck, ears
-dry eyes and throat

77

       -headaches, vertigo
       -aversion to cold
       -sweating palms, face, or chest
       -abnormal uterine bleeding
       -polyuria and nocturia
       -low back weakness and weak knees
       -loss of sex drive
       -fatigue

Tongue: usually pale, possibly with a wet coating
Pulse: Here the pulse could be deep and weak or fine and fast depending upon whether Yin or Yang is more compromised.

## CHINESE PATTERNS AND AMERICAN WOMEN

Modern TCM gynecology texts differentiate menopausal syndrome into the several patterns listed above. However, as previously mentioned, one rarely sees such discrete patterns in individual patients and especially not in American women. Rather, most menopausal American women tend to have some element of Liver Blood, Kidney Yin *and* Yang, Heart Blood, and Spleen Qi Deficiency with Floating Yang in the Upper body and Fluid Dryness in the Lower, all further complicated by Liver Qi Stagnation. Symptoms of all these patterns appear in different combinations depending upon a specific woman's constitution, current stress level, diet, and many other factors. The most common symptoms of this composite pattern are:

       -hot flashes and night sweats
       -palpitations
       -low back pain, possible sciatica
       -irritability and emotional instability
       -fatigue
       -constipation, or alternating constipation and diarrhea

-insomnia
-bleeding gums
-dysfunctional uterine bleeding
-polyuria, nocturia
-loss of sex drive

Tongue and pulse: Because this combination pattern can arise with so many variations it is impossible to suggest only one tongue or pulse conformation.

Once women go through menopause, their consumption of Yin slows down drastically. No longer losing Blood on a monthly basis they cannot really afford to lose, they retrench and consolidate their Yin. If menopause proceeds smoothly and is not allowed to drag itself out, most women have few menopausal complaints and can live another twenty years or more before beginning again to feel marked symptoms of decline. There are many preventive therapies and lifestyle modifications that can help menopause to proceed more quickly and smoothly. Additionally, Chinese medicine offers a number of therapeutic options for women who need professional support during this time. The following chapters describe these preventive and remedial options.

# CHAPTER SIX
# HEALTHY MENOPAUSE:
# A SECOND SPRING

Going through menopause does not automatically mean that symptoms will arise. Just on the physical level, if a woman's diet is good, if she exercises moderately but regularly, if she limits stress in her life where possible and has an effective way of dealing with stress when it does arise, that woman is less likely to experience symptoms when she reaches menopause or at any other time for that matter! There are women who sail through menopause with little or no discomfort whatsoever.

It is important to reiterate that menopause is not a disease. Quite the contrary, it is an intelligent homeostatic mechanism on the part of a woman's body. We have discussed this in earlier chapters but this is such an important and, for Western women, such a novel statement, that it bears review.

As was previously stated, after the age of 35 or so the digestion naturally begins to lose its efficiency. This means the Stomach/Spleen is less able to create Qi and Blood from the refined essence of the digestate. Because there is no long a surplus of Qi and Blood being transformed by the Stomach/Spleen, as time goes by there is less and less Postnatal or Acquired *Jing* to be sent to the Kidneys for storage. Again, this is like capital and interest. If the body is not creating Postnatal *Jing* (interest), it will have to begin dipping into its finite supply of Prenatal *Jing* (capital). This at least partially describes the aging process, but need not necessarily imply disease symptoms.

The Kidneys as well as the Stomach/Spleen begin to decline in function in our late 30's. This will also have a negative impact on the creation of Blood since the Kidneys along with the Spleen and Heart participate in its production. It is said that the Blood and *Jing* share a common source - the Kidneys. This implies that each month when a woman menstruates, some *Jing* Essence is lost with her menstrual Blood. Indeed, the menstruate is the outward physical manifestation of *Jing* in a woman. Once her body is no longer producing a surplus of Blood and *Jing* this situation of monthly loss cannot go on indefinitely if she is to remain healthy. After a certain age menstruation is draining her Kidneys and exhausting the *Chong* and *Ren* Meridians.

At some point the body recognizes what is going on and, to slow down the loss of *Jing* and Blood, shuts down the monthly menstrual cycle. This homeostatic mechanism is the menopause. It is a healthy and positive response of the body to the natural aging process and allows a woman the possibility of remaining in relatively good health with very slow decline for another 20 to 30 years. If there were no menopause, a woman would age much more quickly due to the continual drain of Blood and *Jing* which are the nutritive (Yin) foundation of the body.

Let's now move on to what things a woman can do for herself to facilitate the process of menopause and ensure that it proceeds smoothly and without discomfort.

# CHAPTER SEVEN
# PREVENTION AND SELF-HELP

Menopausal women need not believe that they are doomed to years of hormonal nightmare. Premenopausal women need not anticipate with dread the menopausal years. All women, however, need to act with intelligence to bring their being into a state of health whereby menopausal discomforts may be reduced or eliminated. On the one hand it is important for all of us to recognize and accept the facts of aging and decline. These are part of the human condition and used to be accepted as such. On the other hand, we need not believe that either menopause or the post menopausal years doom us to several decades of excessive and continual suffering. It is up to us to determine how these years will be experienced, and it is up to us to act upon that determination. The following chapters give several suggestions for perimenopausal women to improve their bodies' overall health, increase their production of Qi and Blood, and reduce stress and therefore Liver Qi Stagnation, thereby improving their chances for a healthy and symptom free menopause and slower decline in the postmenopausal years.

Since aging according to Chinese medicine has to do with the state of the Kidneys and since so many signs and symptoms of menopausal syndrome are directly related to decline of the Kidneys, most of the suggestions classically given to perimenopausal women have to do with maintaining the health of the Kidneys. In this book, however, equal attention will be given

to the health of the Liver, which, in my opinion,
is equally important in our culture and at this time in history.
The order in which these suggestions are given does not imply
an order of importance. All of them are important, but few of
us have the time to do everything that is described here as
useful. As you read, note which suggestions you personally
resonate with and can accept or incorporate into your life and
which you cannot, and why. Consider that perhaps the ones
you have the most resistance to may be the most important for
you.

Remember that these suggestions are given with the understanding that not all of them will be or even should be taken.
Few of us are capable of doing everything that we know is
good for us, and moderation even in the things that are good
for us is probably a sign of a relaxed and basically healthy
attitude to life. Try to develop habits or choose regimes that
fit into your life without creating more stress. If you find that
you feel you cannot make any of these options a part of your
life, you may want to think about whether your lifestyle is a
fundamentally healthy one and if some basic changes need to
be made.


## EXERCISE


Everyone needs exercise to maintain health. Exercise is
important for stress reduction, weight control, and cardiovascular health. To be effective for cardiovascular health, exercise
need not be overly strenuous. Studies done recently have
shown that moderate exercise may be just as beneficial to the
heart and lungs as vigorous exercise[20]. Of course, it is also true
that for weight reduction, more calories are burned with more
vigorous exercise or a combination of moderate and vigorous

84

exercise during the same session. But whether you are a vigorous or moderate exerciser, it is, as the advertisement goes, very important to "just do it" and on a regular basis.

If you are not interested in sports, or in joining an aerobics class, many normal daily activities can be exercise. Housework, yard work, walking to work or to the bus stop, washing the car, all these are exercise. If you are really motivated, walking or biking to work has the added benefit of helping the environment and saving money on gasoline, parking, and auto maintenance. If none of these activities are possible on a regular basis, try finding a walking, jogging, or bicycling buddy. This will give you the incentive to keep up your schedule since there is another person depending on you for your support. This also helps prevent boredom since it gives you someone to talk to while you're exercising. However a woman goes about getting sufficient regular exercise, a number of benefits will accrue to her, all of which are valuable.

For menopausal women, regular exercise is even more important because lowered levels of blood estrogen are related to an increased risk for cardiovascular disease in women over 50 years of age. **Exercise has been shown to be of benefit in reducing cardiovascular disease.**

Another continuing issue for many women after menopause which is related to exercise is weight control. Some Western doctors believe that this struggle with weight is related to the fact that the estrogen which our body continues to produce after menopause requires fat cells for its metabolism and use by the body. This increase in fat cells is the body's way of trying to create more estrogen as blood levels of estrogen begin to drop.[21] **Exercise has always been an important part of weight control programs, and can help the menopausal woman**

85

**control this tendency to store excessive fat.**

By this I do not mean that women can or even should try to regain or maintain the figure of a sixteen year old. This is neither a possible nor a healthy endeavor. It may even be true that a body with a *little* extra fat on it is healthier than a very thin one. Remember that from a Chinese medical point of view substance is Yin, and Yin is what most menopausal women are lacking. Excessive or neurotic thinness can exacerbate Yin Deficiency. Too much substance becomes pathogenic Dampness and is also not healthy, but as a culture we often err to the side of trying to be too thin for our own health.

**The third reason why exercise is important is that it helps control stress and minimizes Stagnation.** Stagnation is the opposite of movement, so the external movement provided by exercise circulates the Qi and Blood and any other substance in the body tissues which may be stuck. If the Qi is flowing freely, the emotions are more likely to be balanced and flowing freely as well. If the emotions are flowing freely, there is less tendency for the Qi to Stagnate in the first place. Women with a tendency to irritability, anger, or moodiness will benefit greatly from regular exercise and so will those around them!

Also, from the point of view of Chinese medicine, regular exercise stimulates the Spleen and strengthens the Lungs. Since we know that the Spleen is less active as we grow older, anything which helps the Spleen function will improve digestion, help transform Dampness and Phlegm, and boost the general energy level. Strengthening the Lungs is also important because, according to Five Phase Energetics, it is the Lungs which must keep the Liver in check. This prevents Liver Qi from becoming Excess, rising up out of control, or venting itself on other Organs, most commonly the Spleen and Stomach.

Finally, many studies have been done which show that **weight bearing exercise, even of a relatively moderate type, such as walking, swimming, or dancing, will increase bone calcium levels of post menopausal women, and help prevent bone demineralization or osteoporosis.** Since 90% of all cases of osteoporosis in the U.S. occur in postmenopausal women[22], it is easy to see why exercise is so important. Risk factors for osteoporosis include:

-Caucasian or Asian heritage
-a family history of osteoporosis
-lifelong low calcium intake
-early menopause
-surgical removal of ovaries at a young age
-a sedentary lifestyle
-no children
-excessive alcohol, salt, or caffeine intake
-cigarette smoking
-excessive protein intake
-treatment with steroid drugs
-hyperthyroidism

Obviously, the more of these risk factors anyone has in their lifestyle or medical history, the higher is their risk for osteoporosis, and concurrently, the more is their need for regular weight bearing exercise. Other preventive therapy for risk of osteoporosis will be discussed in the section on orthomolecular or micronutrient therapy and in Appendix II.

For some of us, exercise comes naturally and is not a difficult part of our lives. Unfortunately, it is often the people who resist exercise that need it the most. For example, people with an overabundance of pathological Dampness and Phlegm in the form of overweight find it difficult to exercise energetically. Yet, because exercise mobilizes and melts Dampness and Phlegm, it is a very important part of therapy for anyone with this type of problem. Since the sedentary lifestyle that many women have by this time in life may lead to overweight, regular exercise becomes all the more important. If you are a person for whom the commitment to exercise is difficult to make, try taking it in smaller, simpler steps. Don't create an exercise program that is unrealistic. You will not stick to it and this will just convince your all the more that you cannot do it. Try parking your car closer to home and farther from work or try taking the bus and walking to and from the bus stop. Find a local class in something you've always wanted to learn like tennis, ice skating, or belly dancing. There are also many types of exercise tapes available if you prefer to exercise alone and in the privacy of your home. These can usually be rented from libraries and video rental stores so that you can get an idea of what sort of tapes you like before making any financial commitment. The possibilities for exercise are really limitless. The important thing is that you find something that you like and can stick to on a regular basis.

## STRETCHING

Although stretching is really a type of exercise, I have given it its own section, because it is important for different reasons than those listed above, and because I wish to emphasize its importance. The practice of stretching can be included either as part of an overall exercise program, or as a separate regimen, but it should not be overlooked in any case. In fact, it is my belief that if you cannot discipline yourself to any other type of exercise, stretching may be the most important type of exercise to get.

The reason that I say this is that as we age our bodies become less flexible. This is due to the natural decline of Yin associated with aging. Yin is the Fluid and Blood that keep the tendons, ligaments, bones, and joints supple and flexible. As Yin is lost, there is the natural tendency for these tissues to become dry and stiff. If these tissues are stretched and kept as supple as possible on a daily basis, they will be more likely to remain that way for a longer time.

Additionally, because of this decline of Yin and consequent stiffness, joint and muscle aches and pains are common complaints of older people. Gentle, regular stretching can be a great help in preventing the debilitating effects and financial drain of chronic pain syndromes related to aging.

There are many ways to go about stretching. Most city recreation departments have yoga classes. There are a number of good yoga books and video tapes as well, although if you wish to take up yoga regularly, I suggest taking at least a few classes initially so that you do not injure yourself by wrong postures or overstretching. There are also books available on just plain stretching which are quite good. I have listed several books in the Suggested Reading section which may be of help.

If you are going to aerobics or dance classes, or using exercise videos as your main form of exercise, be sure that there is at least a minimal stretching component to them. One of the healthiest postmenopausal women I know, despite a double mastectomy eight years ago, is a dance teacher who stretches and exercises daily. She is a reminder to me not to underrate the importance of exercise for overall health.

Finally, whatever type of exercise you choose to do, there are a few things to remember:

-Regularity or consistence is more important than vigorousness.
-It is important to pick something that you enjoy doing.
-Regular stretching should be a part of every exercise regime.
-The quality and comfort of your golden years will be directly related to the health of your body.

# ABDOMINAL SELF-MASSAGE

Self-massage may sound strange to some women, but its efficacy for improving health has been known in Japan for centuries. Although there are self-massage regimes for the entire body, the abdomen or *Hara* is considered especially important. In Japanese, the *Hara* is the entire soft portion of the belly. It stretches from just below the diaphragm to the top of the pubic bone. In Asia this area is considered a person's vital center. Anatomically, it contains all the vital Organs of Oriental medicine except the Heart and Lungs. In traditional Japanese medicine, it is believed that a healthy *Hara* is the sign of and key to health in general.

Traditionally, the *Hara's* health is ascertained through palpation (touch). Pain, lumps and bumps, abnormal muscular tension, abnormal pulsation, and hyper or hypotonicity may all be signs that the Internal Organs are imbalanced or dis-eased. A corollary of this is that, if this pain or other abnormal

90

findings are relieved, the imbalance or disease of the Internal Organs these signify will simultaneously be relieved.

Happily, one can not only diagnose the balance and imbalance of the Organs by palpating the abdomen but one can directly treat these Organs and Bowels with nothing more than pressure applied with one's own hands. Many famous Japanese therapists, such as Kiyoshi Kato and Naoichi Kuzome, treat the full range of human disease primarily through *Hara Shiatsu* or abdominal massage.

The Stomach, Spleen, and Intestines are of primary importance to health according to traditional Chinese medicine. If the Stomach and Intestines are functioning normally, abundant Qi and Blood will be produced. Likewise, the Clear Yang (consciousness, intelligence) will arise and the Turbid Yin (waste products) will descend for excretion and evacuation. This rise and descent is called the Qi Mechanism. A healthy Qi Mechanism insures that the Qi and Blood will travel unobstructedly in their proper directions and to their proper destinations, thus nourishing and empowering all the functions and tissues of the organism. When the Qi Mechanism and the Stomach and Intestines are functioning in a healthy way, neither Qi, Blood, Dampness, Phlegm, Food, or Fire will have an opportunity to become Stagnant and thus give rise to disease.

The Intestines or Bowels like to be "empty" according to traditional Chinese medical theory. This means that the Bowels function correctly when they constantly send down the Turbid, the residue, for excretion. When this residue or Turbidity is retained within the organism, it gives rise to numerous disease mechanisms. It is the Qi which empowers peristalsis and moves the Turbid down through the Intestines.

91

Abdominal self-massage is one easy but nonetheless effective way to keep the Qi and Blood in the Internal Organs flowing unobstructedly and the Bowels from becoming Stagnant with retained Turbidity. Although *Hara Shiatsu* is often performed professionally in Japan by trained therapists, it is easy to do oneself and is all the more effective when done on a daily basis.

One begins by lying on their back with their knees drawn up. If the feet are spread slightly apart, the knees can fall together in the center and hold themselves up without any further effort. Next one presses with the flats of the fingers of both hands under the right ribs. One begins pressing as one exhales. Continue to press and exhale to a count of six. When inhaling, move the fingers down and over to the sides of the rib cage and exhale and press again. Do this three times until one winds up pressing under the floating ribs at their sides. See Figure 13 on page 81.

Next go back to the midline beneath the ribs and repeat this sequence moving to the left in three exhalations. During this first pass over the hypochondrium, the pressure should not be too strong. Now repeat this entire sequence two more times, each time pressing a little harder.

At first, it is not uncommon to experience pain, resistance, or tension pressing on this area under the ribs, which is called the hypochondrium, This is a sign of congestion, mostly in the Liver and Gallbladder, which rule this area. As one continues over a period of weeks, this pain and tension will disappear and one's fingers will sink deeper under the ribs. This is quite important because it means that the Liver's main function of governing the smooth dispersal of Qi and Blood is improving. When the Liver's smooth dispersal function is healthy, peristal-

92

sis is normal and digestion is good. Also, one's mood will be even and light and one will have regular elimination and freedom from depression. Therefore, one can see that just this first *Hara Shiatsu* move promoting the free flow of the Liver Gallbladder Qi can have a deeply healing effect.

Next, one positions their hands on their lower right abdomen next to their pelvic bone. With each exhalation, one presses down for a count of six. As one inhales, one moves up the abdomen until finally their hands are beneath the ribs again. One makes three passes up the abdomen on the right side. Anatomically this follows the course of the ascending colon.

Then, beginning at the solar plexus, one presses down the midline to just above the pubic bone. Likewise, one makes three other lines down the left abdomen moving from the center out to the sides. These passes down the left abdomen follow the course of the descending colon. One should repeat this entire sequence up the right and own the left sides of the abdomen three times, each time exerting a little more pressure.

Next, go back to any places where one felt special pain or resistance. As one exhales, exert pressure on these spots to the limits of one's tolerance but without torturing oneself. Often the same spots or areas will be sore day after day. But as one does this abdominal self-massage day by day, these areas will tend to become less sore and sensitive. Typically, in a relatively healthy person, after from two to four weeks of doing this regime daily, one's abdomen will be free from any such specially reactive areas. This signals that incipient Stagnations within the Organs and Bowels have been relieved even before they may have given rise to any other signs and symptoms.

According to some doctors, if one finds an actual lump or mass

93

in the abdomen, besides having this checked by a primary health care professional, one should not press directly on the center of such a lump. Rather, one should search for a sore or sensitive spot on the edge or periphery of the mass. It is here that pressure should be exerted.[23]

Finally, one returns to the right hypochondrium and again presses once three times out to the right and then from the solar plexus once three times out to the left. This concludes one's daily session of abdominal self-massage.

After from two to four weeks of daily practice the average person will find their abdomen has become painless and supple. This should be accompanied by better bowel movements, better appetite, and therefore better, more abundant energy. This entire procedure takes approximately 15-20 minutes. It can be performed directly upon arising or just before bed. After the abdomen becomes pain free and normalized, one can do the massage every other or every few days. However, if one does not take care of oneself, after some time, the pain, lumps, and tension may return and these are signs that one's imbalance has also re-established itself.

In traditional Japanese medicine, it is felt that sensitive spots, lumps, and tension in the abdomen are precursors to more serious disease. A person may otherwise be symptom free but to many Japanese physicians, if there is some abnormality in the *Hara* as diagnosed by palpation, there is some incipient disease process taking shape. Therefore, if one eliminates these abnormalities, one can abort such disease processes even before other signs and symptoms arise.

Also as stated above, ten of the twelve Organs of traditional Oriental medicine are located in and can be accessed through massage of the *Hara*. Also, Meridians connected to four of the most important Organs, the Kidneys, Spleen, Stomach, and Liver traverse the soft abdomen and are directly affected by this abdominal massage.

One cannot easily massage their entire body, but one *can* easily massage their abdomen. Since the abdomen or *Hara* is the Root of the entire body, massaging it massages the Root of all the rest. If the root of a plant is healthy, the leaves and branches will likewise tend to flourish. Although abdominal self-massage appears simple, yet it is based on voluminous and profound theory. For those interested in reading more about the *Hara* and its importance in Oriental medicine and also more about *Hara Shiatsu*, the reader is referred to *Hara Diagnosis: Reflections on the Sea* by Matsumoto and Birch.[24]

# STRESS AND RELAXATION THERAPY

In our culture stress is endemic -- job stress, political stress, environmental pollution stress, relationship stress, sexual stress, travel stress, the stress of the constant decisions required by living in a "free" society. We have created a society which produces more stress than the human body can process and still remain healthy. Past a certain age, most of us will develop symptoms due to this fact. These symptoms may come and go and we can learn to keep them largely under control, but it is arrogant and unreasonable to think that we can forever keep up the often frenetic pace (physically or emotionally) which many of us must ( or believe we must) in order to survive and still be free of the ravages of stress.

Women especially find themselves at a time and place in history with "unlimited" options, where our roles are multiple and our sense of self often ill-defined. Our family structure is weaker and less supportive than at any time in American history; community support for parenting, women's health care, and menopausal issues is inadequate; divorce is endemic; and the stay-at-home mother-and-housewife is no longer an option in most cases. The arrival of menopause is another stressor in and of itself. It brings us face to face with aging, loss of fertility, and possibly the empty nest syndrome. We know that our culture is not supportive of postmenopausal women, and somewhere deep inside this may affect our sense of self worth. The constant demands on the time of the average 35-55 year-old woman in our society often leave us with no "down" time and the feeling of being always behind, always pushed, always squeezed. This is what Stagnation of Qi, specifically Liver Qi, feels like.

The single most important part of any treatment program for symptoms related to Stagnation of Qi is daily relaxation. We have already discussed the fact that the presence or absence of Qi Stagnation may spell the difference between the presence or absence of menopausal symptoms and their severity. This therapy, if done consistently and with perseverance can make a difference on a long term basis, not only in terms of menopausal or other symptoms, but on the fundamental level of who a person is. The reason this therapy is so effective is that it addresses the long term effects of stress and emotional upset, which are at the root of all problems due to Liver Qi Stagnation. In most cases having an emotional component, I believe this therapy can be as beneficial as a good psychotherapy. This is because I believe that whatever happened that makes one frustrated or angry or bitter or afraid is better released and forgotten as quickly as possible. This does not mean that psychotherapy or other counselling may not also be useful in helping us sort out difficult situations in our lives, or that

96

changes may not need to be made, but regular daily relaxation will help us to let go of the things we cannot change and keep even the ones we can change in perspective so that external situations do not put our health in jeopardy.

The emotional responses that we have to  situations are healthy in that they may help us to see that changes need to be made in our lives.  Making changes to improve our life and limit our stress may be difficult.  If our problems are complex, we may need the help of professional psychotherapists, our family, job counselors, our church, or friends. Perhaps for some women major changes are not possible. But no matter how we go about changing our lives or not changing them, holding onto anger and frustration is not useful and it has been demonstrated in both Western and Chinese medicine that it is deleterious to the health. Regular relaxation therapy will help us to do the letting go.

Daily relaxation therapy is one way to turn off the Heat of stress, loosen the vise grip of that squeezed feeling, and lessen the toll that any pressures in our lifestyle can take on our health.  In moments of anger and frustration I find it useful to think of two things. First, consider whether what is making you angry will matter in a year.  If not, then you may be wasting your precious energy being angry.  Second, I try to remember that the best revenge is a good life. Stewing in my anger does not feel like a good life to me.

In order for this therapy to have measurable clinical effectiveness there are a few criteria which must be met.

> 1. It must result in somatic, physical relaxation as well as mental relaxation.

2. It must result in the center of consciousness coming out of one's head and into some part of the lower body, preferably the area of the lower abdomen.

3. It must be done a minimum of 20 minutes per day, although no longer than 30 minutes are required.

4. It must be done every day without missing a single day for at *least* 100 days.

There are many possible techniques which may accomplish this type of relaxation, including hatha yoga, certain types of meditation, biofeedback training, etc. The easiest way that I have found, however, is to purchase one or two relaxation or stress reduction tapes available at health food stores, or "new age" bookstores. These take about 25-30 minutes each, are relatively inexpensive and require minimal discipline.

Some people say that they cannot relax, or that it is very difficult for them to keep their mind concentrated during meditation, or that they do not have time to relax. It is precisely these people who need to relax the most. The tapes are helpful for these people, in that, to some extent, they supply the needed concentration. Each time the mind wanders, the tape brings one back to the task at hand, so that one does not need to concentrate on anything, just to listen to the tape.

Additionally, it is best to try to do the tape at the same time each day, so that after a while it becomes like eating, getting dressed, or brushing your teeth, in other words a nondiscretionary part of your day.

At the end of three months a person may expect to be calmer, less flappable, and have a generally increased state of health with fewer of their prior symptoms manifesting.[25] At the end of three years of regular practice, one will be a different person altogether.


# SMOKING AND RECREATIONAL DRUGS

We all know that smoking is deleterious to the health. From a Chinese medical point of view tobacco is Dry and Bitter and damages the Lung Qi. The Lungs control the Liver, as has been stated several times, and are responsible for astringing the Surface to control perspiration which is very important for menopausal women. Furthermore, the Lungs are the Mother of the Kidneys. If Lung Yin is damaged by the Heat and Dryness of tobacco, Kidney Yin will suffer. It is interesting to note here that smoking is a major risk factor for osteoporosis, and according to Chinese medicine, the Kidney Yin and *Jing* rule the bone and the marrow. Menopausal women can ill-afford to damage the Kidney or Lung Yin.

Recreational drugs come in all types, and therefore have varying effects on the body. None of them, however, is useful for the menopausal woman. By and large they damage the Liver and Kidneys, leading to weakness of both these Organs, the possible deleterious effects of which we have already discussed in detail from many points of view.


# FINDING PURPOSE AND MEANING

In Western culture, as well as in China, up until fairly recently

99

women did not often live into great age.  Many women died in childbirth, from excessive childbearing or overwork, over exposure to the elements, and all manner of diseases.  When we read the classics of Chinese medicine, we can see that a woman of 49 was considered an old woman.

In our century, at least in Western countries, this has changed. Most women have 15-30 good years after menopause in which to work, to contribute, to create.  In fact, there may be fewer stressors on women during those years than there were in the previous two decades, as the duties of rearing children or producing income are lessened, leaving them freer to partici-pate in other activities.  At the same time, most women have, by popular media standards, lost much of their physical beauty and sexual attractiveness by this time in life.  Women must find another source of self esteem and life satisfaction than a good figure or a pretty face.

What I am leading up to here may be the most difficult self-help suggestion that I have, but it is perhaps the most impor-tant since it relates to our mind and Heart.  What I have observed is that the women for whom menopause is the easiest are those women with a purpose larger than themselves in their life.  This purpose may be societal, political, ecological, artistic, or spiritual, but it must be strong enough to short circuit any media or other input from the popular cultural bias which damages basic self esteem.  By this I am not talking about some sort of false ego boosting.  I am talking about usefulness which allows the development of inner strength and inner beauty.  For, if we have not the impermanent beauty of youth, nor the inner beauty which grows naturally from purpose and enthusiasm, it is then that our lives feel empty and mean, and there is room for anger, frustration, and depression.  From a purely medical point of view, it is then that we feel stuck --

100

and feeling stuck is the experience of Stagnant Liver Qi.

Of course this may not be easy and it may even sound trite, but among the people that I know, it is the ones with purpose who seem to be the healthiest. This is not to say that one has to be Mother Theresa, Indira Ghandi, or Jane Goodall to have a meaningful life. Neither is it to say that women with useful, purposeful lives have no health problems. Perhaps, however, if one feels useful, the magnitude of ones problems seem less, and are easier to cope with or rise above.

For some women this suggestion may imply volunteer work; for others it may imply a career change. There are no rules which say what gives meaning to a life. But it is certain that what gives meaning to life can change life for the better, bringing happiness and self esteem in a real sense, which in turn cannot help but be reflected in the health of our bodymind.

Besides the suggestions in this chapter, there are other possible things that a woman can do for herself to help prevent the arisal of disease. An important one that is not included in this chapter is proper diet and vitamin/nutrient therapy. In fact these are so important that the following two chapters are entirely devoted them.

# CHAPTER EIGHT
# HELPING YOURSELF THROUGH DIET

There are people who believe that diet is the major key to health and that all health problems can be solved with a proper diet. After 15 years of work in the field of health care, I am convinced that this is not the case. While dietary advice should always be part of a overall health plan, it is my personal opinion that without proper exercise, no matter what we eat, it will not be digested as well or as completely as it could. Additionally, without proper relaxation, any tendency to Stagnation will be aggravated, which also affects how well we digest our food and absorb nutrients. Nonetheless, our diet can make us sick, and major improvements in health can be made by adjustments in a person's diet. Especially diseases which have a digestive or eliminative component can be greatly affected by specific dietary adjustments.

For women who are perimenopausal, that is women who are nearing, in the middle of, or have just completed menopause, there are certain issues that diet can address and certain Organs whose functions are important and can be supported through good diet. Obviously, the Stomach, Spleen, and Intestines will be either positively or negatively affected by diet. This in turn will have an indirect but nonetheless important effect on the Liver, Kidneys, Lungs, and Heart. In fact, there is a lineage of Chinese medicine which came from a famous doctor, Li Dong-yuan (1180-1251 C.E.), who based his entire treatment of the body and all its tissues and Organs on rectifying the diet and digestion.[26]

Certainly there is solid Chinese medical theory to back up Dr. Li's ideas. If the Spleen and Stomach are healthy, there will be abundant Qi and Blood production with a concomitant increase in Postnatal *Jing*. This, in turn, will retard the aging process by supporting the Kidneys and not requiring them to use up Prenatal *Jing* for basic metabolic processes. Also, an ample Blood supply assures the Heart and Liver of adequate Blood allowing them to house the Spirit and Psyche comfortably. This ensures better sleep and emotional health. In fact, treatment of the Spleen is an accepted method of treatment for Liver disorders in general, even in acupuncture or herbal medicine.[27]  Also, if the Spleen is healthy, it will not draw excessively on the Kidneys, which are the pilot light for the Spleen/Stomach which are, in turn, the "burner" responsible for the combustion of nutrients. Additionally, according to Five Phase theory, the Spleen(Earth) is the Mother of the Lungs (Metal). Therefore, if Earth is healthy, it can create Metal, allowing the Lungs to flourish. This then results both in good Heart function and the natural control of the Liver.

There are many foods and ways of eating food which support the health of the Stomach/Spleen. These include:

> -eating mostly foods which are cooked and warm
> -eating foods which are easily digestible
> -eating mostly grains and vegetables with small amounts of meat and meat broths
> -avoiding or limiting cold, frozen, and raw foods
> -limiting foods which produce Dampness, such as milk products, especially if there is a tendency to

produce mucous
-using cautiously the warming spices such a ginger,
    cardamom, nutmeg, and cinnamon which benefit
    the digestion

Concerning cooked versus raw food, there has been a great
deal of literature touting a raw foods diet as being the way to
health. This is based on the presumption that raw foods have
higher levels of vitamins and minerals which can be destroyed
in cooking. However, while some cooking processes can be
destructive to certain vital nutrients, what this idea fails to
consider is how the digestive process actually works. Digestion
is a process of combustion. The Stomach must make everything that goes into it into 100 degree soup before anything
else can happen.    Anything which helps the Stomach by
partially pre-digesting food, such as the process of cooking, will
help the Stomach do its job more efficiently and with less
effort. This, in turn, allows the body to absorb the available
nutrients more efficiently. Raw foods require more work from
the Stomach. Even lightly steaming or stir-frying aids the
digestive process without harming most nutrients. Furthermore, if the nutrients which remain in cooked food are more
absorbable than those in raw food, the net effect is improved
nutrient absorption. Also, if the Stomach does its job well the
Spleen, which is the next Organ down the line in terms of
digestion and energy production, will be more likely to do its
job well. Consider further that one does not give raw foods to
a sick person or to a baby, but rather cooked foods which are
more easily digestible, therefore imparting strength for
recuperation or for growth.

The basic traditional diet that humans have thrived on for
several millennia is a combination of cooked grains, whole, in
noodles, or in breads, beans or legumes, vegetables (usually

105

cooked) and fruits in season with small amounts of dairy and meat. Even modern weight loss diets such as the Pritikin program are based on this same combination. The reason that this diet works for weight loss is that it supports the Spleen and Stomach which automatically keep the body from accumulating Dampness and Phlegm, i.e. fat.

Concerning Dampness and Phlegm, there are several foods which create Dampness in the body -- dairy products, excess meat, nuts, oils, and sugar. While small amounts will not cause problems in most people, when eaten to excess these can cause pathogenic accumulation of Dampness. This in turn interferes with proper Spleen function, decreasing the Spleen's ability to transform Phlegm and Dampness, and to create enough Qi and Blood. This is a vicious circle which can lead to many other problems. For example, it is said that though the Spleen is the creator of Phlegm, the Lungs are its home. This means that Phlegm may lodge in the Lungs leading to upper respiratory dysfunction. Phlegm may obstruct the Meridians, where it may cause numbness, paralysis, lumps, nodules, or tumors. Finally it may obstruct the Heart where it disturbs the Spirit, causing behavioral changes, madness, or unconsciousness. Dampness, which is a slightly different entity from a technical Chinese medical point of view, can cause stiffness of the joints, sluggish movement, heavy limbs, fuzzy thought processes, or turbid, cloudy, sticky secretions or excretions. Considering all the problems that pathogenic Dampness or Phlegm can cause, foods that contribute to their accumulation should be limited.

Concerning the caveat against frozen foods, these are even harder for the Stomach/Spleen to process and are rather like dousing a precious fire with ice water. Again remember that the Stomach must bring all foods up to body temperature before they can be digested and you can see how much harder it is for frozen and cold foods to be digested. Also we must consider that up until 40-50 years ago there was no refrigeration and frozen foods did not really exist. While refrigeration is a great gift for keeping food fresher longer, it is questionable whether or not we should eat foods straight out of the freezer or refrigerator. Any food will be easier to digest at room temperature. As for ice water, it tastes great on a hot day, but should probably be drunk between meals so as not to slow down digestion thereby leading to Stagnant Food and/or Dampness.

The mild warming spices, most of the basic pumpkin pie spices if you noticed, give a mild boost to the movement of Qi and slightly invigorate the Stomach without the damage that can be done by strong Qi movers such as caffeine and heavy pungent spices such as cayenne pepper and jalapenos. These are fine to include in the diet in judicious amounts as long as they do not aggravate Heat symptoms such as hot flashes or night sweats.

While the Liver is more deeply affected by emotions than by diet, there are foods which can aggravate an imbalanced Liver, and should be avoided. These include:

-coffee including decaff, and other caffeinated foods
    or beverages
-alcohol, except in small, infrequent amounts
-greasy, fried, or oily foods
-spicy, pungent, hot dishes such as curries or chilies
-excessive meat consumption and other hard to digest
    foods such as nuts and beans
-chemicals, pollutants, and preservatives

Lets go over these one by one. Caffeine, especially in the

107

form of coffee (and even decaff), is not a food according to Chinese medicine. It is used as a drug, and in small doses. Its functions are to strongly activate the Qi and bring the energy from the core of the body to the surface. The activity of Qi has to do with the consumption of Yin by Yang. Therefore, by strongly activating the Qi, a certain amount of Yin and Blood (substance and fluid) will be used up. This exhaustion of Yin and Blood skews the relationship between Yin and Yang which in menopausal women is already precarious at best. The net effect of long term caffeine consumption is, therefore, extremely deleterious to a woman's health most especially at this time in her life. Of course, if a woman suffers from any symptoms of Liver Qi Stagnation, she will really like the kick which the caffeine gives to the Qi and may have a terrible time overcoming the habit. While the caffeine temporarily frees up the movement of the Qi, it will eventually waste the Blood. Since the Liver Blood is what allows its Qi to flow unobstructedly, the entire situation is actually exacerbated in the long run. If a woman can make only one change in her diet, slowly weaning herself of coffee (including decaff) and other forms of caffeine is probably the best dietary change that she can make for her health.

Alcohol in small amounts from time to time relaxes the mind and makes for social conviviality. Its energetic nature is, however, Damp and Hot. When used to excess it overheats the Liver and Stomach, and dampens the Spleen. Since Dampness weakens the Spleen and Excess Heat injures the Blood and exacerbates any tendency to Heat symptomology, we can see that neither of the attributes of alcohol is useful for a menopausal woman. In short, one should keep their consumption to an occasional beer or glass of wine.

In addition to Dampening the Spleen, greasy or oily foods tend

108

to clog the digestive mechanism. Their frequent consumption can lead to Food Stagnation and Spleen Dampness. Also, it is the Liver/Gall Bladder which is responsible for the metabolism of fats through the creation and secretion of bile. Over consumption of these foods creates excessive work for the Liver, which, like an engine running for too long, will tend to become overheated.

Spicy foods have a similar effect to that of caffeine. Most of us with Liver Stagnation will be drawn to them as they give a kick to the Liver Qi. However, because the Pungent flavor relates to the Metal Phase according to Five Phase Theory, its excessive consumption will tend to weaken the Lungs, whose job it is to keep the Liver in check. Additionally, since this flavor is inherently Hot and Dry in nature, it will overheat the Liver and Stomach and dry the Blood. In any disease which has an element of Qi Stagnation, the consumption of pungent foods is classically forbidden.[28]

This book does not tout vegetarianism. Although meat need only be eaten in small amounts or in the form of broths, it is probably important for most people to include a small amount of it in their diets, because it is an excellent food for preventing Qi and Blood Deficiency. On the other hand, large quantities of it are difficult to digest, produce pathogenic Dampness, and are unnecessary for adequate protein consumption. Soups made from meat broths or marrow bones are an excellent way to get the most nourishment from meat without the part which is hard to digest and unnecessary for health.

The effects on our food supply of preservatives and other chemicals or pollutants found in the soil and water is known to be deleterious to the health. Many of these substances are carcinogenic or toxic to various organs. While it may not

109

always be possible to buy organically grown food, it is advisable to do so as much as possible.  Especially as we get older, our bodies are less able to neutralize or excrete these substances and it is advisable to eliminate them as much as possible from our diet.  Also, by demanding more organically grown foods we are sending a message to the retailers, the food growers, and to the government bodies with which they interact.  This will eventually have the effect of increasing support for organic farming methods.  As the supply of organic foods increases the prices of these foods will come down.

Finally, this discussion has spoken of the effect of diet on other Organs leaving out the Kidneys.  While the Kidneys are affected by the health of all the other Organs, it is also possible to treat the Kidneys directly through diet.  It is said in the Ling Shu, Chapter 36 that "the *Jing* extracted from the five cereals reaches the bones and nourishes the brain and marrow."  Since bones, marrow and brain tissue are the outgrowth or flourishing of the Kidney *Jing*, this passage is referring to the nourishment of the Kidneys.  By using the term five cereals there are two implications.  One is that all the five flavors of Five Phase Theory will have an effect on the Kidney, and that the consumptions of grains specifically is tonifying for the body in general.

In classical Chinese dietary theory, grains should be partially processed or polished which makes them easier to digest.  This is interesting in light of the fact that, according to Western nutritional biochemistry, excess bran and fiber from grains creates an excess of phytic acid in the body inhibiting the absorption of calcium and other minerals into the bones, again bringing us back to the Kidney *Jing*.

Other foods which are specifically good for the Kidneys are

110

soups made from marrow bones, walnuts, lotus seeds, grapes, pork and turtle meat, chicken, actual kidney meat from sheep or ox, potatoes, and pears.

If Liver Yang is hyperactive with Heat symptoms in the upper body, foods which lower Yang include barley, beef broth, asparagus, apples, bananas, lettuce, and celery.

Foods which calm the Spirit include rice, oyster, longan fruit, wheat and wheat germ, and many types of mushrooms.

One Organ that we have left out of this discussion on diet is quite important. The Large Intestine will be greatly affected by diet. The Large Intestine receives the Impure or Turbid part of the foods which we eat. From this it extracts the "Pure" part from the Impure and, via an Internal Channel, this is sent to the Kidneys. This is the process by which the *Wei* or Protective Qi which we discussed in several earlier chapters is created. While it is the Lungs which control the *Wei* Qi, it is the Large Intestine and Kidney which create it. If the Qi mechanism of the Large Intestine is overstuffed due to Food Stagnation or if the motility of the Large Intestine is stuck due to Liver Qi Stagnation, the Large Intestine will not remain open and its function of discharging the Impure and its role in creating *Wei* Qi will be hindered. If the Impure waste products remain in the body they can cause a number of problems.

From a Western physiological point of view this problem can lead to auto-toxemia whereby the waste products in the large intestine begin to putrefy and send poisonous by-products back into the body via the blood. Furthermore, the large intestine houses many friendly bacteria which participate in the body's immune response. Proper intestinal health is very important is preventing or treating immunological disorders and improving

**111**

immune response.

From this discussion it is easy to see why diet and nutrition is so important for maintaining good health, and especially when the body is going through the delicate balancing act of menopause. To make this even more specific, let us go on to look at specific nutrients which are important during menopause and why.

# CHAPTER NINE
# SPECIFIC NUTRIENTS
# FOR A HEALTHY MENOPAUSE

All of the micronutrients, by which I mean vitamins, minerals, amino acids, enzymes and coenzymes, are important for the maintenance of good health. There are, however, several that are more important than others at the time of menopause and beyond for maintenance of the Organs and tissues of the body both from a Western and Chinese medical point of view. This chapter gives both a Western nutritional and Chinese energetic rationale for the importance of these specific nutrients in the diet of women in general and of menopausal and perimenopausal women in particular.

Many people say that they would rather get their vitamins and minerals from food sources and not take supplements. This is understandable since good supplements are expensive and also require a person to remember to take them. Unfortunately, with our food and water being largely contaminated, our soil depleted, and our stress levels so abnormally high, most of us probably need supplementation with extra vitamins and minerals more than what we can get from food.[29]

## VITAMINS

Without vitamins the foods we eat can not be utilized by the body. Vitamins facilitate the biochemical reactions by which food is used for energy, repair, and all metabolic functions. The food itself is the raw material upon which the biochemistry of the body acts to do this and vitamins are catalysts between the raw material or food, and the enzymes. Without vitamins enzymes cannot act upon food to create energy.

From a Chinese medical or energetic standpoint we can describe each vitamin as if it were a Chinese herbal medicinal. Each one acts as either a tonifier, regulator, disperser, or nourisher of various energies, Organs, or tissues in the body. As such the practitioner of Chinese medicine can use them similarly to herbal medicine for various energetic imbalances. Unlike herbs, however, vitamins are absolutely necessary in minimum quantities to maintain health.

**Vitamin A** tonifies the Blood, benefits the *Jing* Essence, brightens the eyes, nourishes the Skin, clears Heat from the Blood, and treats Deficiency Fire Patterns. Since hot flashes and night sweats are usually signs of a Deficiency Fire condition, adequate vitamin A is important for menopausal women. We have also discussed at length the importance of Blood and *Jing* to menopausal health.

Vitamin A is an important vitamin for the lubrication of the mucous membranes of the body, including the mouth, nose, urinary tract, vagina and external genitalia, and the eyes. It also plays a role in bone and teeth formation by assisting the absorption of calcium. A deficiency of it can lead to night blindness, retarded growth in children and dry, scaly, painful mucous membranes. Since we know that bone demineralization and vaginal atrophy or dryness are important issues for post menopausal women, it is important to ensure an adequate amount of vitamin A in the diet.

**114**

Vitamin A is found pre-formed in animal foods such as fish oils. Remember when our mothers doled out spoonfuls of cod liver oil? Doses of pre-formed vitamin A should be kept to no higher than 25,000 units per day. Vitamin A, however, does come in another, safer form. It can be synthesized in the body from its provitamin, Beta-carotene. This is the substance which gives orange and yellow color to many fruits and vegetables. Although masked by green chlorophyll, it is present in large quantities in deep green leafy vegetables as well. It is also present in large amounts in dairy products.

It is wise to get as much as possible of our vitamin A from food sources such as green and orange vegetables and fruits, since many supplement forms of the vitamin include high amounts of retinol or retinyl palmitate which is not water soluble and can build up in liver and fatty tissues of the body to toxic levels. Since cooked green and yellow vegetables should be included in the diet daily, it should not be difficult to get enough in the diet. For example, the MDR (Minimum Daily Requirement) for an adult is 5,000 IU (International Units) and a cup of cooked carrots has 15,000, half a fresh cantaloupe has 9,000, and a cup of cooked broccoli has 4,500.

**Vitamin B$_1$** regulates the Qi, activates the Qi, strengthens the Spleen, dries Dampness, helps prevent Stagnation, expedites the free flow of Liver Qi and stops pain.

**Vitamin B$_2$** tonifies the Blood, nourishes & tonifies the Liver & Kidneys, treats Deficient Yin & Blood Patterns including *Lao Bing* and Wasting Disease, nourishes Stomach Yin, and benefits the *Jing* Essence.

**Vitamin B$_3$** relaxes constrained Liver Qi, harmonizes the Liver/Stomach, Liver/Spleen, clears Heat from the Stomach,

115

and raises Yang Qi.

**Vitamin B<sub>5</sub>** regulates the Qi, relieves Liver Qi Constraint, harmonizes the Liver/Spleen/Stomach, raises Clear Yang, clears & eliminates Damp Heat, and clears Heat from the Liver.

**Vitamin B<sub>6</sub>** clears Heat from the Liver/Gallbladder, extinguishes Wind, harmonizes Wood & Earth, relieves depression, and clears Heat from the Stomach and Damp Heat from the Gallbladder.

**Vitamin B<sub>12</sub>** tonifies the Qi, tonifies the Qi to transform the Blood, and stops bleeding.

**Vitamin B<sub>15</sub>** regulates the Qi, activates the Blood, disperses Stagnation, and benefits the Heart and, therefore, indirectly the Lungs.

**Biotin** nourishes the Blood, relaxes the Liver, nourishes the Skin, tonifies the Heart Blood, and calms the *Shen* Spirit.

**Choline** nourishes the Blood, extinguishes Wind, nourishes the *Jin* Sinews, and moistens the Intestines.

**Folic Acid** nourishes the Blood, relaxes the Liver, calms the *Hun*, and secures the Fetus.

**Inositol** nourishes the Blood, moistens the Intestines, Nourishes the Skin, and calms the *Hun*.

**PABA** tonifies the Liver & Kidneys, tonifies the Blood, benefits the *Jing* Essence, moistens the Intestines, promotes bowel movements, expels Wind from the Skin, blackens the hair, and retards aging.

116

From a Chinese medical point of view, looking over the B vitamins as a group it is easy to see that they are important especially for nourishing the Blood and Kidneys, regulating the Liver, and calming the *Shen* (Spirit) and the *Hun* (Psyche). Specifically for menopausal women, $B_5$ is useful for fatigue, constipation, and digestive disturbances suggesting that it harmonizes the Liver and Spleen. PABA nourishes the Blood, skin, and *Jing* Essence, and is useful for keeping the hair from greying, preventing constipation, and easing irritability.

It has long been known in Western nutrition that stress depletes the B vitamins as a group, and that people with a high stress lifestyle need higher doses of the B vitamins as a group to maintain a healthy nervous system, sound sleep, and strong blood. In relationship to menopause specifically, PABA and $B_5$ (Pantothenic Acid) are known to have positive effects on vaso-motor disturbances (hot flashes and sweating), and $B_{12}$, Folic Acid, Biotin, and Inositol have a calming, soothing effect on the nervous system. To discuss in detail the positive effects of each of the B vitamins could take volumes.

**Vitamin C** clears Heat, stops bleeding, clears Heat and dissolves Toxins, clears Heat from the Heart, and calms the *Shen*. This is why it is effective in the treatment of colds, flues, and various infections, which, according to Chinese medicine, often tend to be of a Hot or Warm nature. Since hot flashes, irritability, insomnia, night sweats, and headaches are commonly due to rising Deficiency Heat in menopausal women, adequate dosage of vitamin C is obviously useful. In relationship to dysfunctional uterine bleeding, if the cause of the bleeding is Heat in the Blood layer, then vitamin C can be useful as a styptic in these situations.

According to Western biochemistry, vitamin C is useful for

**117**

menopausal women because of the high metabolic demand for it by the adrenal glands in situations of stress. The adrenal glands are responsible for the production of estrogens when the ovaries are no longer capable. The adrenal steroid androstenedione is converted to estrone. Vitamin C is required for this process. Interestingly, in Chinese medicine, the functioning of the adrenal glands is related to Kidney Yin which is typically Deficient in menopausal and post menopausal women. Additionally vitamin C is required in order for the body to absorb calcium into the bones. It is important to note that vitamin C needs to be in a pH buffered and electrolyte and mineral balanced form to increase absorption, reduce the risk of diarrhea, and decrease urinary loss.

**Vitamin D** tonifies the Kidneys, benefits the *Jing* Essence, mends the Sinews & Bones, brightens the eyes, and calms the Fetus. All of these functions, with the exception of the last, are important to menopausal women and even more so during the post menopausal years.

Vitamin D controls blood levels of calcium and phosphorus and oversees the process of bone mineralization and calcium excretion from the kidneys. If there is inadequate vitamin D, calcium cannot be absorbed by the bones even if enough of it is available. While there is no MDR of vitamin D for adults, the best source of it is sunshine which allows the body to synthesize it internally and store it in the liver. While we all know the dangers of too much sun exposure, it is important to get enough for the body to store vitamin D for the cold months when the skin gets little exposure. Even 10 or 15 minutes a day in shorts and a t-shirt is plenty, longer if the body is only partially exposed.

**Vitamin E** tonifies the Yang, nourishes Liver Blood, tonifies

118

Kidney Yang, benefits the *Jing* Essence, and nourishes the *Jin* Sinews. This vitamin is important for keeping the Liver and Kidneys nourished and strong. Since many of the musculoskeletal complaints of older people, including osteoarthritis, are due to Liver Kidney Dual Deficiency, this vitamin is extremely important for anyone over 40 as a preventive therapy. Since Liver Kidney Deficiency is the dominant mechanism of aging, vitamin E can be seen as an age retardant.

Vitamin E (Alpha-Tocopherol) functions as an antioxidant in unsaturated oils. That means that it is a scavenger of destructive substances in the cell membranes which are related to the aging and break down of the cells. In relationship to menopausal symptoms, multiple studies done earlier in the century showed that effective vitamin E therapy can control severe hot flashes in more than 50% of cases.[30] This means that women should be sure to get adequate vitamin E, probably starting well before they reach menopause. Vitamin E requirement increases at menopause and if a woman decides to do estrogen replacement therapy, her need for vitamin E is even greater.[31]

The most abundant source of vitamin E is unsaturated vegetable oils such as sunflower, safflower, walnut, and wheat germ. Whole grains are also a good source. Both sources, however, can be damaged or destroyed by rancidity, so proper storage without freezing is important. Also, the less an oil is refined or processed, the more intact remains all its vitamins, including vitamin E.

**Vitamin K** stops bleeding, astringes the Intestines, contains leakage of Lung Qi, and restrains leakage of Blood. This vitamin is important for women with problems such as dysfunctional uterine bleeding.

119

Vitamin K is synthesized by the healthy bacteria in the intestines, so once again we can see the importance of healthy intestine ecology. Women who are at risk are usually ones with a history of recent or continual antibiotic therapy which destroys the healthy bacteria which colonize the intestine. Vitamin K is necessary for the production of prothrombin, a chemical required for blood clotting. It is also found in green leafy vegetables, yogurt, egg yolks, and blackstrap molasses.

**Bioflavonoids** regulate the Blood, clear Heat, stop bleeding, and clear Heat from the Liver. For women with a tendency to Liver Stagnation and Heat symptomology such as rib and flank burning or pain, premenstrual syndrome and irritability, or painful, fibrocystic breasts, the inclusion of supplemented bioflavanoids is appropriate.

Bioflavanoids are important in female biochemistry because they increase capillary tone similarly to how estrogen affects capillary tone. When estrogen becomes less abundant, it is important that the estrogen receptor cites on the capillary walls have another substance with which to bond to maintain capillary tone, this substance being plant flavonoids. It is the capillary tone which helps control vasodilation or vasoconstriction of the blood vessels. This in turn can have a great effect on whether a woman experiences hot flashes and night sweating.

**Beta-carotene** activates the Qi and dredges the Liver, clears Heat and dissolves Toxins, disperses Stagnations and Accumulations, and combats cancer. Since the risk of cancer increases with age and markedly after menopause, it is important for all women over 40 to make sure they get enough of this substance.

Beta-carotene is believed to stimulate the thymus to produce

120

T cells which are necessary part of the immune system for the elimination of infection. Life span studies in Japan following 250,000 people over a 10 year period showed that a diet high in Beta-carotene decreases risk of lung, colon, stomach, prostate and cervical cancers.[32]

# MINERALS

While 96% of the body's weight is made up of oxygen, hydrogen, carbon, and nitrogen, the other 4% are collectively referred to as minerals.  Despite their small percentage of body make up, they are vitally important to health.  They are found as constituents in all the cells, enzymes, hormones, and in many of the vitamins, and especially within the hard tissues of the body such as teeth and bone cells.  Further, the ionization of minerals into electrolytes is what allows for the positive and negative electrical charges which permits the flow of an electrical impulse along the nerves.  Many of the minerals are absorbed through the intestinal walls which again reminds us of the importance of a healthy intestinal environment for so many metabolic functions.

Similar to vitamins, Chinese medicine can describe the energetic functions of the minerals, thus allowing them to be used preventively and remedially.  While all the minerals are important, only the ones especially important for perimenopausal women are discussed below.

**Calcium** settles and calms the *Shen*, benefits the Yin and restrains Floating Yang, absorbs acid and stops pain, descends Yang and extinguishes Wind, clears the Liver and brightens the eyes, strengthens the Bones and promotes the generation of new tissue.  This mineral is useful therefore to improve sleep, stop or control aches and pains in the joints and muscles, and benefit Heart, Kidney, and Liver Yin.

According to Western biology, Calcium is the most abundant mineral in the body. It acts in cooperation with phosphorus to build and maintain bones and teeth. With the help of magnesium, it is also essential for regulating the heartbeat, preventing insomnia, and for healthy blood. Calcium also helps maintain proper blood pH levels and participates in muscle contraction and nerve transmission. Deficiency of this mineral initially shows up as twitches, muscles cramps, nervousness, irritability, or numbness in the arms and legs. Serious deficiencies are seen in cases of osteoporosis, osteoarthritis, loose teeth, and severe tremors. Calcium absorption decreases with the decreased production of estrogen beginning as menopause. It is known that exercise of a weight bearing nature (where muscles pull against the bones to which they are attached) is useful for keeping adequate levels of calcium in the bone and preventing osteoporosis. See Appendix II for a more complete discussion of calcium and mineral absorption in general.

**Chromium** tonifies the Qi, tonifies the Spleen and benefits the Qi, and tonifies the Qi and Blood. This mineral is useful for improving the Spleen's function of creating adequate Qi and Blood and transforming Damp. It is therefore useful for women with a tendency to become fatigued easily or to accumulate Dampness in the form of fat as is common during menopause.

Biochemically, Chromium stimulates the activity of the enzymes involved in the metabolism of glucose (sugar) into energy, and for the synthesis of fatty acids and cholesterol. It is an important substance for the maintenance of proper blood sugar levels and to prevent wild swings in appetite. Since it is difficult to absorb, it is important to get it in foods from which it is most biologically available such as brewer's yeast, liver, beef, whole wheat, beets, and mushrooms. Women with severe appetite swings or the tendency to binge on sugar may find a supplement of chromium picolinate to be useful.

**Copper** drains Dampness, promotes urination and leeches out Dampness, strengthens the Spleen, and clears and eliminates Damp Heat. This mineral seems to be related to the Spleen's function of ruling the flesh and keeping it elastic and firm.

Western nutrition indicates that copper is useful in keeping the hair from greying because it helps convert the amino acid tyrosine which in part give pigment to the hair and skin. It also aids the body in the formation of elastin, the chief component of muscle fibers. It also assists in the production of the myelin sheaths which protect nerve fibers. Copper is relatively easy for the body to absorb and is found in sea food, whole grains, almonds, leafy green vegetables, and beans, depending upon the copper levels in the soil where they are grown.

**Fluorine** tonifies the Kidneys, nourishes Yin, and strengthens the bones and teeth.

Fluorine is a trace mineral necessary for the deposition of calcium in the bones. It comes in two forms, sodium fluoride, which is often added to water supplies to combat tooth decay, and in its more natural form of calcium fluoride, which is found in seafoods, meat, and cheese. It is easily absorbed by the body and in fact is highly toxic if too much is absorbed in the form of sodium fluoride. If it exceeds 2 parts per million in water supplies it is antagonistic to many important metabolic functions. See Appendix II for a fuller discussion.

123

**Iodine** clears Heat, clears the Liver, and dissipates Nodulations. It has been effectively used in remedial dosages to treat breast lumps caused by Heat and Stagnation of the Liver.[33]

Iodine is described in Western nutrition as necessary for thyroxin production by the thyroid gland.   Since thyroxin supplementation is common for menopausal women with fatigue problems, iodine is an important mineral at this time. Further, iodine has been shown to be effective in reversing fibrocystic breast disease.  It is easy to get adequate amounts through dietary sources such as seafoods (both animal and vegetable) or sea salt.

**Iron** clears Heat and cools the Blood, nourishes the Yin and Blood, invigorates and dispels Congealed Blood, and clears Deficiency Fire and Ascendant Fire.  These functions of iron indicate its importance for menopausal women in preventing hot flashes, headaches, night sweating, abnormal bleeding, irritability, and insomnia.  Iron helps the Blood to carry out its function of nourishing the muscles, Organs, and all body tissues.

Iron is found in every cell of the body and always is combined with protein.  Its major function from the Western medical point of view is to combine protein with copper to create hemoglobin, the substance which makes a red blood cell red and is responsible for transporting oxygen from the lungs to all the tissues to prevent disease and create resistance to stress. It is an important mineral at all times in a woman's life. However, its usage in the body increases during menstruation, pregnancy, lactation, or whenever there is a loss of blood. Women with fibroid tumors causing excessive bleeding often develop iron deficiency related anemia.  To be absorbed, all forms of iron must be converted to a form called ferrous iron.

The iron that is in the body is reused many times and only small amounts of the iron in use is excreted from the body. This is good because 90% of all iron ingested is never absorbed by the blood.

Animal foods are by far the best sources of iron, with liver topping the list. Leafy green vegetables, whole grains, dried fruits, some beans, and molasses are also fair sources. Excessive consumption of caffeine inhibits iron absorption as does a lack of hydrochloric acid in the stomach.

**Magnesium** settles and calms the *Shen*, benefits the Yin and restrains Floating Yang, prevents leakage of Fluids, and absorbs acidity and stops pain. This is a very important mineral for women with insomnia, muscular tension, anxiety, or irritability.

Magnesium is necessary for many vital metabolic processes. It is necessary inside the cells for the metabolism of carbohydrates and amino acids. As the counterpart of calcium it plays an important role in neuromuscular contraction and relaxation. It also assists the body in the absorption of other minerals, including calcium, and vitamins C, E, and B complex. Adequate amounts of it are therefore vital for a healthy menopause. Also, since the risk of heart disease and severe coronary thrombosis increases greatly after menopause, magnesium is needed because of its preventive effect on these diseases. It also helps reduce blood cholesterol and prevent nervous disorders. Blood levels of magnesium in alcoholic persons are usually found to be very low.

Being an essential element in chlorophyll, magnesium is found in all green vegetables, as well as in dairy products, seafoods, soybeans, whole grains, and oil-rich seeds and nuts.

125

**Manganese** nourishes the Yin and benefits the *Jing* Essence, nourishes the *Jin* Sinews and strengthens the Bones, and benefits the hearing. Its effect on the Kidneys is seen by the fact that a lack of adequate manganese leads to tinnitus and hearing loss. In Chinese medicine hearing is controlled by the Kidneys.

Western medical sources indicate that a deficiency of manganese can lead to diabetes since is plays a vital role in glucose tolerance levels in the blood. Severe deficiencies can lead to hearing loss and dizziness, which are not uncommon in older people.

**Phosphorus** tonifies the Kidneys, nourishes the Yin, benefits the *Jing* Essence, nourishes the *Jin* Sinews, strengthens the Bones, and promotes the healing of the *Jin* and Bones, all of which functions are important during menopause.

Phosphorus is the second most abundant mineral in the body and is found in every cell. It functions with calcium to insure the maintenance of the bones, and these two minerals must remain in proper balance to be effectively used by the body. There are few chemical reactions in the body in which phosphorus in not required. Fortunately phosphorus is easily absorbed through the intestine as long a there is an adequate supply of vitamin D and calcium. It is stored in the bones and teeth, body phosphorus content being regulated by urinary excretion. Good dietary sources of it include all animal protein products, whole grains, seeds, and nuts.

**Potassium** drains Dampness, promotes urination, strengthens the Spleen, stops diarrhea, clears Heat and expels pus, expels Wind Dampness, and clears and eliminates Damp Heat, including Damp Heat in the Liver/ Gallbladder. This mineral is especially important for women with Spleen weakness manifesting as fatigue, loose stools, water retention or easy weight gain.

Potassium works with sodium to regulate water balance within the body, normalize the heartbeat, and nourish the muscles. According to Western scientific research, a potassium deficiency can cause nervous disorders, insomnia, muscle weakness and exhaustion, water retention, and heart arrhythmias. It is easily absorbed in the intestines and can be found in all vegetables, grains, oranges, bananas, and potatoes, especially the skin.

**Selenium** benefits the Yin, restrains Floating Yang, settles and calms the *Shen* Spirit, astringes the *Jing* Essence, and brightens the eyes and relieves superficial visual obstruction. This mineral has a similar energetic effect as many other minerals, although it is only required in trace amounts in the body. It appears to retard the aging process of the Kidneys and Liver.

Although only small traces of selenium are required in the body, it is an important antioxidant, neutralizing harmful effects from toxic compounds which would otherwise interfere with the immune response to invading microorganisms. Since immune response weakens as we age, this mineral is even more important in our diets after 40 than before. Selenium is abundant is organ and muscle meats, dairy products, brewer's yeast, fish, and grains.

**Sulfur** nourishes the Blood and the Liver, nourishes the Skin, blackens the hair, cools the Blood, and benefits the Skin. Since the Kidneys are responsible for the pigment or lack of pigment in the hair, this substance must have a positive effect on the Kidney *Jing* Essence.

127

Often called nature's beauty mineral due to its positive effect on the skin and hair, this nonmetallic element occurs widely in nature and makes up one quarter of one percent of body weight. It is necessary for healthy nerve and liver tissue, and makes the hair glossy and the skin smooth. Sulfur hot springs have been used for centuries by people all over the world to soften the skin and relax the muscles, but sulfur is not found in abundance in plant foods. Eggs are the best food source with some also being found in meats, fish, and dairy products.

**Zinc** benefits the *Jing* Essence, nourishes the Blood, strengthens the Bones, brightens  the eyes, and tonifies the *Jing* Essence to check Evil Qi. Because of its effect on the Blood and *Jing*, like other minerals, zinc is important for slowing the aging process, mostly of the Kidneys.

Fortunately, a balanced diet of mostly unprocessed foods should be zinc sufficient. However, zinc can be depleted by stress, alcohol, or an unbalanced diet. Zinc is important because it facilitates the absorptions of the B vitamins and is a component of at least 25 enzymes involved in digestion.

Most of us probably need at least a multiple vitamin/mineral supplement to maintain good health, especially during menopause. It is probably best to have a health care practitioner help you decide whether a multiple vitamin/mineral is sufficient, or whether you need extra support from one or more other specific supplements. There are many good multiples on the market, but there are just as many less effective brands. Again, professional advice is probably a good idea. The next chapter on professionally administered therapies discusses some specific vitamin/mineral supplements including multiples and several single or combination supplements which are specifically targeted for menopausal and post menopausal women.

# CHAPTER TEN
# PROFESSIONALLY ADMINISTERED THERAPIES PREVENTIVE & REMEDIAL

Self care is an essential part of any comprehensive health care plan. Indeed, it may be the largest and most important part. There are times, however, when it is appropriate and necessary to seek out the support of professional health care providers. The reasons may be either preventive, remedial, or both. If you are a menopausal woman with symptoms that are more than a slight annoyance, it is probably wise to seek out professional care. Estrogen replacement therapy (ERT) is the most common therapy given to menopausal women by Western medical practitioners and for some women it is no doubt appropriate. (See Appendix I for a more complete discussion.) Chinese and other more natural medicines offer other remedial and preventive options for symptomatic and asymptomatic menopausal women which may be preferable for many.

If you are menopausal and taking estrogen replacement therapy (ERT) but would like to stop, Chinese herbal medicine, homeopathic medicine, and/or specific vitamin/mineral therapy may be able to help you. If you are in your late 30's or early 40's and have any menstrual irregularity, PMS symptoms, fibrocystic breasts, excessive bleeding, or cramps, not only can Chinese herbal medicine, vitamin therapy, and acupuncture help you with your current problems, but by doing so may help you have an easier, less symptomatic menopause. If you are a woman who has passed menopause, who is not on ERT, is planning to stop ERT, or would like to stop ERT, there are other options to keep your bones strong, maintain cardiovascular health, and/or to deal with other potential health problems.

Before describing possible professional therapies in more detail, it seems appropriate here to speak a little about the practice of Traditional Chinese Medicine (TCM) and acupuncture in the United States. Classically, Chinese medical practitioners in China as well as the U.S. limited the scope of their practice to acupuncture, certain types of massage, and herbal medicinals which came from China and were described in the Chinese herbal texts. Most practitioners in China even today are only trained in one of these fields. For instance, an acupuncturist in China does not prescribe herbal medicines, and vice versa. However, the practice of Chinese medicine in America, and indeed worldwide, is undergoing rapid evolution. A major part of this evolution involves the use of medicinals other than those found in the classical texts. As I mentioned in the chapter on vitamins and minerals, the use of any substance as a medicine by a TCM practitioner requires only that the substance be able to be described accurately in TCM energetic terms. A great deal of research is currently being done in the U.S. and other countries to describe vitamins, minerals, Western and other non-Chinese herbs, and even Western synthesized prescription drugs according to these parameters. As this research progresses, more Western practitioners of Chinese medicine will have available a wider range of treatment modalities than did the previous generation of practitioners.

130

Of course most acupuncturists are not legally able to prescribe Western prescription drugs, but it is very useful for them to be able to understand these substances with their own theory and rationale since many of their patients are taking prescription pharmaceuticals at the same time as they are receiving acupuncture or herbal medications. A clear understanding of Western pharmaceuticals from a Chinese energetic point of view allows the practitioner of Chinese medicine to make more informed choices about other therapies which will not conflict with the effect of the drug(s) being taken, nor cause any unwanted side effects.

The areas into which many Chinese medical practitioners are expanding quite rapidly are the use of vitamin/mineral supplementation, sometimes called orthomolecular therapy, the use of non-Chinese herbal medicinals, and the use of homeopathic remedies. While this research and expansion of treatment possibilities is growing, by no means all practitioners of acupuncture or even Chinese herbal medicine are using all of these treatment modalities. Because Chinese medicine has only been widely recognized and practiced in this country for a little over a decade, the range of practice (and legality) in the U.S. is quite wide. Many practitioners only use acupuncture, or acupuncture and massage; others use only Chinese herbs with acupuncture; still others use acupuncture with homeopathy, which is also popular in Europe. All of these and still other combinations may be very effective. However, for the consumer this diversity may be a bit confusing. If you seek out an acupuncturist or a practitioner of Chinese herbal medicine, it is important to ask what his or her range of practice includes. If you are interested is a specific type of therapy, make sure in advance that the person you see practices that therapy.

As the profession of acupuncture/Chinese medicine grows in the West, and as more people are interested in it and other alternative therapies, the scope of practice will probably continue to grow and change. In the meantime, it is important that consumers be as informed as possible about what therapies are available to them and which ones are most effective in which types of situations. In this chapter we will outline several professionally administered therapies which may be of special help to menopausal women.

## MASSAGE THERAPY

Massage is one of the most ancient of healing arts. Its applications are as diverse as the styles currently available. What all massage has in common is the ability to move the Qi and Blood manually. This means that massage in most any form is good for Qi Stagnation problems. Since these kinds of problems are all too common in the West, almost everyone can benefit from regular professional (or even non-professional) massage. Remember that Qi Stagnation can change a symptom free menopause into a quite uncomfortable menopause. Massage has the added benefit of providing emotional nurturance through touch which is not something which our culture in the U.S. has supported and which everyone needs to be healthy. Furthermore, because pain is usually due to something which is Stagnant i.e. Qi, Blood, Dampness, etc., massage can also relieve pain to a great extent by removing the Stagnation and bringing fresh Qi and Blood to the painful area. Finally, from a Chinese medical point of view, because massage is usually very relaxing to the body as a whole, it can have a similar effect as regular daily relaxation by allowing the person to just let go of everything for the hour or so that she is on the

132

table.

There are two basic types of massage that need to be discussed -- oil and non-oil massage. They are not equally useful for all women, largely due to the nature of the oil itself.

In the section on dietary therapy we spoke of oil as having a Damp energetic nature. For women who are already too Damp internally, those who are overweight, sluggish, easily fatigued, or with a tendency to chronic oozing or weeping skin lesions, oil massage is probably not the best choice. This is just adding Dampness to Dampness, and while the woman may enjoy the massage, there are other better options for her body type.

Oil massage is good for women who are hyperactive, workahol-ic, thin, wiry, always on the go, and find it difficult to relax or rest, possibly with a tendency to insomnia. Earlier in this book we discussed Wind in the body and how it creates incessant, involuntary movement. In some ways women with this second profile have a type of Wind disease -- they are always moving, rarely still. The oil has the effect of dampening the Wind, smoothing it out and slowing it down. There are several types of oil massage available around the U.S. It is probably best to find a practitioner with a good reputation and get a few massages from different practitioners to find one that you like the best.

For women who are of a more phlegmatic, slow moving nature, non-oil massage forms are probably a better choice. Japanese massage, often called *Shiatsu, Anma*, or *Amma*, Chinese remedial massage, called *Tuina* (pronounced tway-na), and Tragger massage, are all possible choices. These forms of

133

massage are usually done with the person clothed and often work with the same theories of Meridians and Organs as an acupuncturist uses.

There are many other types of massage/body work which can benefit menopausal women including Reflexology, Sports Massage, Rolfing or Structural Integration, *Jin Shin Jyutsu* or *Jin Shin Do,* Therapeutic Touch, and Neuromuscular Massage. Most of these will be good for moving Stagnant energies, providing the nurturance of touch, and allowing the woman to relax, lie down, and be taken care of. The more vigorous, deep muscle therapies such as Rolfing and Neuromuscular massage may not be as relaxing in process but can help women with chronic musculoskeletal pain in many cases.

Beyond the dichotomy of oil or non-oil massage, a woman must consider the importance of finding someone with whom she feels comfortable and with whom she can relax. Also, there is the issue of what type of massage is available in one's area. If you are interested in receiving massage even occasionally, you'll need to find a well trained massage therapist. You can find out if there is a school of massage therapy in your area. If so, they may have a public massage clinic for their more advanced students which offers massage for quite reasonable rates. They will also probably have a list of graduates, where they are practicing, and in what kind of massage they specialize.

It is also a good idea to ask other health care providers if there are any capable massage therapists to which they could refer you. You may find that your acupuncturist, physician, or chiropractor has a massage therapist to whom they refer on a regular basis or even one who works in their office.

If the yellow pages are your only source of information, look over the advertising carefully to see if the person states anything about their training or is a member of one of the many massage therapy organization, such as the American Massage Therapy Association (AMTA), the Associated Professional Massage Therapists (APMT), the On Site Massage Association (OSMA), or the California Health Practitioner's Association, all of which require certain educational standards for membership.

You may think that massage is such a simple therapy that it cannot possibly make any profound metabolic or organic changes. It is my experience, however, that this is not the case. There are volumes of case histories in China and Japan and ever-growing research in the U.S. which support regular massage therapy for most stress related ailments, such as insomnia, headaches, digestive disorders, PMS, and many others. Like anything else, however, in order for anything profound or deep to happen, you have to stick with it for a while. If this sounds like something you could include in your life on a regular basis, it comes highly recommended with several millennia of recorded clinical history behind it.[34]

# ACUPUNCTURE

Acupuncture is also an ancient healing art. Its recorded practice goes back more than 2000 years, and the literature upon which it is based is voluminous. While its applications are broad and its efficacy well documented, acupuncture is not the most important and effective modality for many menopausal complaints. This has to do with the concept of Excess and Deficiency.

135

If you think back upon the earlier chapters of this book which discussed the theories of Chinese medicine and explanations of menopausal symptoms, most of the signs and symptoms of menopause have to do with Deficiency. Even in cases where there is an Excess, it is often only a relative Excess, existing only because of an underlying Deficiency. The most common of these Deficiencies are of Yin or Blood or both. Qi and Yang can also be Deficient, but these are less common situations.

Acupuncture is the insertion of needles into the body at specific points. It works by moving the Qi and by releasing or breaking up Stagnation in the Channels and Collaterals. The movement of Qi is similar to the movement of electricity, and acupuncture works like a system of breaker switches, sockets, or on and off buttons to facilitate the movement of Qi, Blood, Yin, and Yang over the Meridians of the body. However, acupuncture can only move energies which are already present in the body. It is not very good at supplementing energy which does not already exist. That is, it is not a modality which is effective for adding to or tonifying a significant Deficiency of a particular energy. At best it can only catalyze the creation of such energy through the stimulation of one Organ or another.

The use of needles, however, is only half of the practice of acupuncture. In Chinese, the word for acupuncture is *Zhen Jiu* which translates as needle and moxibustion, or simply moxa. Moxibustion is the practice of burning the herb Artemisia Vulgaris Sinensis, a common sage family herb, on under, over, or around the acupuncture points or other areas of the body. While this practice does in fact add energy to the body and is used in Deficiency situations, this energy is in the form of

136

Heat. Since many, even most of the common symptoms which arise with menopause involve an element of rising Heat caused by Deficient Yin, adding more Heat must be done with great care, if at all. There are some practitioners who may be able to use moxa in Deficiency Heat situations with skill and success, but this is a delicate process and can cause exacerbation of symptoms if not done properly. If, on the other hand, a woman has the pattern of Kidney/Spleen Yang Deficiency with cold limbs, aversion to cold, diarrhea, fatigue, and Organ prolapse, without much in the way of Heat signs and symptoms, moxibustion may be quite effective in alleviating her symptoms.

Despite these limitations, certain symptoms may be brought under control more quickly with acupuncture therapy as part of the overall treatment plan. These include palpitations, uterine bleeding, and night sweats. Also, acupuncture may be helpful at relieving symptoms which are specifically due to Stagnation of Liver Qi such as mood swings, excessive sighing, distention and pain in the abdomen, chest, sides, or upper back. On the other hand, regular relaxation therapy is often even more effective and less expensive for Qi Stagnation problems than acupuncture, although a combination of both can have dramatic effects.

Except in specific cases, our clinic does not usually recommend acupuncture as the therapy of choice for patients with menopausal complaints since herbal and orthomolecular supplementation is typically so effective and especially if used in combination with minor dietary and lifestyle adjustments as discussed in the previous chapters.

# HERBAL THERAPY

Herbal medicine is one of the most effective natural methods of treating menopausal complaints or preventing their arisal. Many single herbs and herbal preparations have been and can be used in cases of menopausal discomfort. Most of them will have at least limited success in relieving the basic menopausal symptoms of hot flashes, night sweats, and insomnia. All of them have varying applications depending upon the specific pattern or combination of patterns being treated. In Chinese medicine, herbs are rarely used singly. Most formulas, whether prepared as a powder, pill, tincture, or tea are a combination of from six to twenty herbs.

Herbs are effective in cases of Deficiency because they actually add energy to the body. Furthermore, herbs work largely through the medium of the Blood and Yin, unlike acupuncture which mostly manipulates Qi. Since most menopausal health issues relate to the Blood and Yin and to Deficiency, herbs are an appropriate choice. Herbs have the added advantage of being whole and biochemically complex substances made up of a balance of various synergistic chemical parts. This means that they are easier for the body to utilize than single, synthesized drugs, and that in turn means they are less likely to cause side effects.

However, such freedom from side effects is based on correct administration in turn based on a correct professional diagnosis. This is why it is usually a good idea not to self-medicate. Do not make the mistake of thinking that since herbal medicines are natural substances, herbs are completely benign. The wrong herbs or the wrong dosage can make a person sick or worsen their health. So if you are seriously interested in taking herbs for preventive or remedial menopausal care, it is wise to seek professional assistance in choosing the appropriate formulas.

The following several classic Chinese formulae are used for menopausal and post menopausal complaints. Some of them originated over 1000 years ago. I am listing these to give readers some idea of Chinese herbal medicine. These formulas should only be prescribed, however, by qualified professional practitioners of TCM.

> **Zhi Bai Di Huang Wan** or Zhi Bai Ba Wei Wan is a famous formula  used to nourish Yin, tonify the Kidneys, and control flaring up of Fire due to Yin Deficiency. It is often used as a base formula to which other herbs are added.

> **Da Bu Yin Wan** (Big Tonify Yin Pills) is a formula is often used for menopausal disorders of which a major component involves Blazing or Flaring Fire symptoms, such as hot flashes, headaches, or night sweats.

> **Tian Wang Bu Xin Dan** (Celestial Emperor Tonify Heart Powder) is a formula which nourishes Heart Yin and is strongly tranquilizing and sedating to a disturbed Spirit. It therefore is often used in cases of insomnia.

> **Zuo Gui Wan** (Gathering/Returning to the Left Pills) tonifies the Liver and Kidney and replenishes Yin and Blood. This is often used for post menopausal women with  more Kidney weakness than Deficient Fire symptoms.

**139**

**Er Xian Tang** (Two Immortals Decoction) is a famous formula for menopausal complaints, developed at the Shu Gang Hospital in Shanghai. It is especially effective for cases of erratic periods, because it regulates the *Chong* and *Ren* meridians.[35] It has ingredients for Dual Kidney Liver Yin Deficiency with Flaring Liver Yang and Deficient Kidney Yang as well (both Hot and Cold symptoms).

**Gui Pi Tang** (Restore the Spleen Decoction) has a soothing, nourishing effect on the Spirit and Heart as well as invigorating the Spleen and replenishing Qi. It is a good formula for excessive bleeding due to Deficient Qi during the early part of menopause.

**Ba Wei Di Huang Wan** (Eight Flavor Rehmannia Pill) is for situations of Deficient Kidney Yang where the Kidneys need to be warmed. This formula is contraindicated in cases of Kidney Yin Deficiency, where Yang floats upward causing Heat symptoms but can be used in cases of Dual Kidney Yin and Yang Deficiency.

These formulas are often prescribed in the form of decoctions. That means the herbs themselves are dispensed and taken home to cook in water. This is the most common method of administration in China and is also commonly used in the U.S. This method allows for the formula to be modified with the addition of other herbs which can address specific symptoms. However, it is often difficult to convince a busy career woman with already too much to do and too little time that this is the best method for her. Therefore, many of the above formulae come in pill form or powder form, either from mainland China or Taiwan and with growing frequency from U.S. manufacturer's as well. Pills have the advantage of ease of administration and the disadvantage of not being capable of modification. Sometimes two pill formulae will be given in tandem when one pill does not deal with all the symptoms effectively.

This brings me to the discussion of one particular pill that has been designed specifically for Western women who are approaching or experiencing menopause. This formula is manufactured in the U.S. by a company called Health Concerns and it addresses the complicated pattern of disharmony most Western menopausal patients display as described above. It is called **Damiana and Gotu Kola Two Immortals Tablets.** It is based on the formula Er Xian Tang listed above plus another formula called Er Zhi Tang (Two Extremes Decoction) but has been modified to be more specific for what is seen most often in Chinese medical clinics in the U.S.

It was mentioned in the chapter about patterns of disharmony that while the patterns explaining menopausal syndrome are described as discrete entities, in clinical practice one does not see such discrete patterns in real life patients and especially not in American women. Rather, most menopausal American women tend to have some element of Liver Blood, Kidney Yin *and* Yang , Heart Blood, and Spleen Qi Deficiency with Floating Yang in the Upper body and Fluid Dryness in the Lower. Plus, there is typically the added complication of Liver Qi Stagnation. Damiana and Gotu Kola Two Immortals Tablets include ingredients for each of these issues, which is to say that it was designed for the typically complicated menopausal syndrome seen in American women and is meant as a whole to treat a wide range of menopausal signs and symptoms. These include hot flashes and night sweats, depression, anxiety, irritability, palpitations, low back pain, tinnitus, insomnia,

141

constipation, breakthrough and dysfunctional uterine bleeding, bleeding gums, and even greying of the hair. It can also prevent the occurrence of menopausal migraines and hypertension and can help to prevent breast malignancies.

This formula as well as the others listed above can be prescribed by any practitioner of Chinese herbal medicine when appropriate to an individual woman's situation. They are not, however, panaceas which can or should be taken without professional diagnosis and prescription.

Single herbs can be purchased in health food stores. Two of the most popular for menopausal women are Dang Gui (Dong Quai and Tang Kuei are also alternate spellings) and Ginseng. While these have been shown to be of help in minimizing hot flashes, the dosages at which they are available over the counter in health food stores is probably not adequate unless ingested in large amounts. Also, there are many types of Ginseng on the market. Each of them has a different therapeutic application and taking the wrong one can worsen one's condition. Again, while these herbs may be helpful for menopausal symptoms, it is probably best to take them under the care of someone trained in their use and proper preparation.

Valerian, scullcap, passion flower, chamomile, and hops are also popular Western herbs which are often used to replace stronger, prescription sedatives which may be prescribed for women with insomnia or night sweats. These herbs are usually available in bulk and pill form at health food stores and may also be prescribed as part of a larger herbal formula by Chinese or Western herbalists.

For post menopausal women who are concerned about

cardiovascular disease and osteoporosis, there are also herbal preparations which can be taken over a long period of time to address the patterns underlying these problems. Both cardio-vascular disease and osteoporosis are related to Yin Deficiency in general and Kidney Yin Deficiency specifically. Remember that it is Yin which is the substance or stuffing, the density in the bones. It is also Yin which makes things in the body such as arteries and veins supple and elastic. Accordingly, some herbal formulas, notably Liu Wei Di Huang Wan or Six Falvored Rehmannia Pills, are used by older people in China over a long period of time to tonify Yin and therefore help keep the bones strong and the cardiovascular system supple. There are also several formulas in Chinese herbal medicine specifically designed for keeping bones strong. However, many of these contain animal by-products taken from endangered species. For this reason it is my preference to use vitamin/mineral supplementation as described below for long term therapy such as may be needed to prevent osteoporosis.

# ORTHOMOLECULAR
# (VITAMIN/MINERAL) THERAPY

As stated above, it is probably prudent for all of us to take a good multiple vitamin due to the effects environmental degradation have on our food supply, and the ravages of excessive stress have on our bodies. Research suggests that it is almost impossible to get all the vitamin/mineral substances we need from our foods. A ten state evaluation of nutrient deficiency done by the U.S. Department of Agriculture in the late 1960's showed that large portions of the population are receiving significantly less than the minimum recommended daily allowances of many important nutrients. A more recent

143

study done from 1978 to 1980 found that the problem had actually gotten worse.[36] What these studies indicate is that significant segments of the population are deficient in at least some vitamins, notably the B complex, as well as iron, calcium, and magnesium, if not other minerals as well.

From the findings of these studies the hypothesis can be made that most of us do not have a well balanced and vitamin mineral rich diet. The inclusion of at least a good quality multiple vitamin/mineral supplement in order to maintain adequate levels of these micronutrients is prudent, especially as we age and our bodies are metabolicly less efficient. There are, of course, many good natural brands of vitamins on the market which are free of chemical additives, binders, etc. While many MD's may not prescribe a specific brand, most alternative health care providers will be able to advise you on which companies' products are reliable.

Although there are a number of companies which manufacture similar products, in this book I will refer mostly to the Metagenics Inc. line of supplements. I like their products because they have a very good selection of specific products for women's health care, several of which are excellent for menopausal and post menopausal women. They also manufacture a wide range of other diagnostically specific products as well as a good multiple vitamin/mineral supplement (Multigenics [TM]), all of which are available only through qualified health practitioners. In addition, Metagenics helps ensure that their products are prescribed correctly through various seminars and workshops and voluminous research reprints.

For women with hot flashes and night sweats, Metagenics has a product called Fem-Estro[TM]. This formula is a blend of vitamins, organic glandulars, and herbs which support enzyme production for the balanced metabolism of hormones. It also includes natural anti-oxidants which help protect cell membranes by reducing free radicals. Research indicates that free radical production in the body is a prime factor in aging. This makes anti-oxidants an important part of any age retarding program. This product can be taken for a number of years without side effects and has been used as an effective substitute for estrogen replacement therapy. While only one case of reported side effects is on record after four years of sale, Metagenics suggests that women at a high risk for hyperestrogen related problems, such as certain types of breast cancer, should not take this supplement.[37]

From a Chinese medical point of view, Fem Estro™ is effective for menopausal complaints because it replenishes both Yin and Yang, clears floating Heat, nourishes Liver Blood and Kidney Yin, benefits the *Jing* Essence, regulates Stagnant Liver Qi, and calms the Spirit. This means that it effectively addresses many of the possible disease mechanisms for menopausal complaints.

According to Western nutritional theory, the nutrients in this formula regulate vasomotor function, block the destruction and deactivation of estrogens by the liver, support the adrenal glands which are responsible for estrogen production as the ovaries' production declines, and strengthen capillary walls which helps prevent flushing, and increases overall estrogen production. Its indications include a family history suggesting a tendency to osteoporosis, hot flashes, vaginal dryness, or other clinical symptoms of menopause.

Another product which may be of help for menopausal women

with dysfunctional uterine bleeding is Metagenics Fem-UBF™. This is a formula designed to treat uterine bleeding which, from a Chinese medical point of view is due to Depressive Liver Heat, a common progression of Stagnation of Liver Qi appearing in middle-aged women. Since the Western medical treatment of this problem often includes D and C (dilatation and curettage) operations, or even hysterectomy, many women may want to first try less heroic measures such as Fem-UBF™ first. We have used the product in our clinic with positive results in a number of cases.

Metagenics also has a formula which is helpful for women with fibrocystic breast disease and/or breast pain. This formula, called Fem-FBS™ can be used for pre and well as post menopausal women and should be taken in conjunction with a multiple vitamin/mineral supplement.

There are three other areas of concern for menopausal and post menopausal women which can be effectively addressed by vitamin/mineral therapy. These are osteoporosis, osteoarthritis and related joint problems and anti-oxidant therapy for age retardation.

While much of the current literature on osteoporosis discusses briefly the use of calcium supplementation and exercise for the prevention of osteoporosis, the Western medical community as a whole is quite committed to the use of ERT as the main effective therapy for preventing bone demineralization. For women who do not wish to do ERT or for whom ERT is contraindicated, there is a relatively new product on the market which has proven quite effective in supporting bone tissue and preventing bone mass loss. It is called microcrystalline hydroxyapatite, a substance which helps bones absorb and

146

retain adequate calcium and other minerals to remain strong. Taken in small but regular doses with the proper mineral balance, this substance has been shown to be capable of preventing osteoporosis. Metagenics Inc. sells this substance in two balanced mineral formulas, Cal-Apatite™ and Osteogenics™. For a more complete discussion of these formulas as well as other types of Western therapy for osteoarthritis, see Appendix II.

For women with a family history of osteoarthritis or who have any tendency to degenerative joint disease, there are collagen promoting formulas such as Metagenics' Collagenics™ which has excellent research supporting its use for reversing these types of diseases. This formula is far superior to taking anti-inflammatory drugs, either steroidal and non-steroidal, which, while relieving pain, are also known to cause an increase in the breakdown of connective tissue which is what joint tissue is made of. In the long run, formulas which rebuild joint tissue taken in conjunction with natural, non-destructive anti-inflammatory herbs and bioflavonoids are a better choice in most cases.

The purpose of anti-oxidant therapy is to scavenge free radicals in the cells. Free radicals are toxic by-products formed during the metabolism of fats. They damage protein molecules and DNA and RNA, the basic stuff of which living, healthy cells are made. When cells are damaged by free radicals their breakdown is part of the process of aging. Damage from free radical production can be greatly reduced by antioxidant nutrients such as Beta-carotene, vitamins C, E, bioflavonoids, and the minerals zinc and selenium. Vitamins $B_1$, $B_5$, and $B_6$ are also anti-oxidants, but are best taken as part of a multiple because they are interactive and absorb more effectively in an

147

integrated formula. Most vitamin companies have specifically anti-oxidant formulas with varying amounts of different nutrients. One Metagenics anti-oxidant formula is called Oxygenics™ and is a complete and well balanced anti-oxidant formula. You may wish to consult a health professional before purchasing a specific combination for long term use.

Some women have asked me when it is preferable to use herbal medications and when vitamin/mineral supplements are more effective. There are no hard and fast rules here. What I do find, however, is that for some women, the idea of herbs is a bit too exotic and that they relate more readily to taking vitamin/mineral supplements. For extreme situations such as severe night sweats, severe, recurrent hot flashes, and menorrhagia or uterine bleeding, herbs work quickly and well to alleviate symptoms. However, it may not be cost effective or convenient to keep the client on strong herbs for long periods of time, especially if those herbs have to be cooked fresh each day. In most cases of menopausal syndrome a combination of herbs and vitamin/minerals works best. In our clinic we have used the combination of Metagenics' Fem-Estro with Health Concerns' Two Immortals Tablets to good effect and find it well accepted by patients and relatively cost effective. When further combined with some self-help therapies and a bi-weekly massage, most menopausal women may expect to remain symptom free.

# CHAPTER ELEVEN
# FINDING A PRACTITIONER OF TRADITIONAL CHINESE MEDICINE

Traditional Chinese medicine is a rapidly rising star within the American alternative healthcare community. As of this writing, there are more than twenty American schools and colleges of acupuncture and Chinese medicine. That means that the number of professional American practitioners of this art is growing by about five hundred practitioners per year. Many American practitioners have also either gone to medical school in Asia or have gone to Asia for post-graduate training. And, of course, many Asian doctors have immigrated to the United States in the last twenty years.

In addition, there is a National Council of Acupuncture Schools and Colleges which helps to over-see and regulate the quality of training and education, a National Commission for the Certification of Acupuncturists which helps to insure minimum, entry level, professional competence, and various state and national professional associations, such as the American Association of Acupuncture and Oriental Medicine, which help to regulate professional ethics, network amongst practitioners, and provide continuing, post-graduate education. Acupuncture has now been legalized as a state-approved healthcare modality in over a score of states and in many others, favorable legislation is in the process of being enacted.

In states where acupuncture is licensed and state regulated, one should be able to find the names of local practitioners in the yellow pages of their phone book or by contacting their state Department of Health, Board of Medical Examiners, or Department of Regulatory Agencies. In such states, it is wise to insure that potential practitioners are, in fact, state licensed. In states without licensure, it is best to seek out those practitioners who are nationally board certified. Such practitioners typically append the initials Dipl. Ac., for Diplomate of Acupuncture, after their names. These national board exams insure minimal professional competency and not less than the equivalent of two full years of academic and clinical training specifically in acupuncture.

In the United States, not all acupuncturists are practitioners of Chinese herbal medicine, but almost without exception, all American practitioners of Chinese herbal medicine are also acupuncturists. As yet, only a handful of states include Chinese herbal education and examination in their licensing and, until now, there is no national herbal board exam. Therefore, it is important to query potential practitioners on the school, nature, and extent of their Chinese herbal training. In general, the practice of Chinese internal or herbal medicine is more demanding and requires more education and experience than the practice of acupuncture. Hopefully, in the near future, there will be some kind of national credentialing of traditional Chinese herbalists.

When searching out a qualified and knowledgeable practitioner, satisfied, word of mouth referrals are important. Therefore, it is also appropriate to ask for references from previous patients treated for the same problem. Likewise, it is important that the practitioner be able to communicate with the patient in order to explain their Chinese diagnosis and the rationale behind their treatment plan. In all cases, a professional practitioner of Chinese medicine should be able and willing to give a written traditional Chinese diagnosis of the patient's case. Also, I personally suggest that patients select practitioners who belong to both local and national Chinese medicine/acupuncture professional associations. Such associations offer referrals of professional members in good standing and high repute. In addition, such associations almost always have a code of professional ethics which their members promise to uphold and this further insures the quality and professionalism of the care they provide.

Traditional Chinese medicine, including acupuncture, is a discrete and independent healthcare profession. It is not a technique to be added to the bag of tricks of some other profession. It takes just as long *or longer* to learn Chinese medicine and acupuncture as it does to learn allopathy, chiropractic, naturopathy, or homeopathy, and previous training in one of these systems in no way confers *a priori* competence or knowledge in Chinese medicine or acupuncture. Therefore, I heartily advise prospective patients seeking to avail themselves of the benefits of traditional Chinese medicine to seek out professionally trained practitioners of this system. As suggested above, just as one would not hire a plumber to do electrical wiring, so patients should receive Chinese medicine from professionally trained practitioners of Chinese medicine.

For further information regarding the American practice of Chinese medicine and acupuncture and for referrals to local professional associations and practitioners, prospective patients may contact:

151

National Acupuncture Headquarters
Washington, D.C.
(202) 265-2287

This is the joint offices of the American Association of Acupuncture and Oriental Medicine, the National Commission for the Certification of Acupuncturists, and the National Council of Acupuncture Schools and Colleges.

*"Do not wait for leaders. Do it alone, person to person."*

*Mother Theresa*

# CONCLUSION

Menopause represents a definite reorganization of energies and priorities within a woman. When this change proceeds smoothly, there are minimal complaints associated. But some women seem to get hung up in mid-process. For whatever reason, their Blood and/or Yin have become so weak that even after the crisis triggering the shutting off of the menstruation, they cannot replenish their Blood and Yin as quickly and as easily as other women. Therefore they experience prolonged Yin and Blood Deficiency symptoms and Floating Upward of Yang. These symptoms include hot flashes, night sweats, irritability, hysteria, insomnia, palpitations, vertigo, tinnitus, Heat in the Five Centers (palms of the hands, soles of the feet, center of the chest), forgetfulness, hypertension, low back pain, possible migraines, and depression. While the Deficiency of Yin and Blood which brings the menopause may be inevitable, it is Stagnation of Liver Qi and its complications which prevent the quick recuperation of Yin and Blood that healthy women should experience. Liver Qi Stagnation may be triggered by psychoemotional stress and poor diet.

While we cannot deny or halt the aging process which brings us to this cusp called menopause, there are many things which we can do to facilitate a smoothe passage and to support a healthy aging process without the risks inherent in hormonal or other Western medical therapies. We can eat better, exercise regularly, and learn to manage or limit the stress in our lives as much as possible. What may be even more important, we can take steps to find more meaning and purpose in our existence. From a philosophical/spiritual point of view that is what the second half of life is about -- dealing with our existential dilemma and eliminating the meaningless from our lives. A woman who's life is full with purpose is less likely to be troubled by menopausal complaints and less likely to become bitter over her loss of youth.

This is not to deny or belittle the sexism and agism in our culture. It exists and we must confront it, ignore it, or bow to it. However, simply by our sheer numbers as the "baby boom generation" we have the possibility of recreating in our own unique way the respect, status, and integration that older persons have in some other cultures. As a group now coming into power, we have the possibility to make history, to halt environmental degradation, to tame technology for peace and humanity, and to reintegrate our culture and, thereby, ouselves. Perhaps I am an incurable optimist, and in no way do I wish to minimize the problems that we face as a culture or as a planet. I do, however, believe that my generation of women can be, indeed must be, a major part of the solutions to those problems if indeed solutions are to be found. By so doing, we may find a second spring, the strength and purpose that we need to live whole and healthy through menopause and beyond.

# APPENDIX I
# ESTROGEN REPLACEMENT THERAPY:
# PROS AND CONS

## HISTORY OF ERT USE

By far the most common therapy given to menopausal women for all complaints is estrogen replacement therapy (ERT). This therapy involves the oral, cutaneous patch, or vaginal cream administration of estrogen in order to replace the estrogen which the ovaries stop producing. Usually oral estrogen is given in combination with progestin or progestogens for at least part of the month in order to minimize some of the possible side effects of unopposed estrogen therapy such as increased risk of endometrial growths or cancer. What this combination of medications does is to prolong the youthful hormonal state of women well past their reproductive years. Some women take ERT into their 70's.

ERT has gone through many changes in the last several decades. Estrogen therapy was first used in the 1920's for women who has lost their ovaries. It became quite fashionable in the early 60's for menopausal women to take estrogen and the sales of estrogens quadrupled over the next 10 years. By the early 70's as many as 22 million prescriptions per year for estrogen therapy were being written for menopausal and post menopausal women.[38] Women wanted ERT because they were told they would age more slowly, look better, and avoid the discomforts of menopause at the same time. Also, the drug companies have had a lot to gain by touting estrogen therapy as a larger proportion of our population reaches middle age.

However, by the mid 70's a great deal of research began to appear linking estrogen use with increased rates of endometrial or uterine cancer. At that point the use of estrogen therapy

155

dropped rapidly for several years. In recent years, however, it has been discovered that the use of progestins (a relative of progesterone) in combination with estrogen taken for at least part of the month seems to negate this risk. The progestin allows the uterine lining to be shed at the end of each month much like a small menstrual period. This prevents a build up of the uterine lining which can lead to uterine cancer. In light of this, ERT is now more popular than ever.

## ERT THERAPY OR NOT?

While this therapy is an increasingly popular one, questions about its long term risks have not all been answered. Although adding progestin to the estrogen cycle reduces the risk of uterine cancer, some studies have linked progestin, like the progesterone in birth control pills, to an increased risk of high blood pressure, heart disease, high LDL cholesterol, and stroke.[39] Other studies indicate exactly the opposite, that the use of ERT which includes progestin for part of the month greatly reduce the risk of hardening of the arteries, high cholesterol, and heart disease.[40] Still other doctors state that ERT combined with progestin, calcium, and sodium fluoride could be used safely for the prevention of osteoporosis in most women.[41] Clearly, despite the enthusiasm that some doctors show for ERT, there are unanswered questions even from a Western medical standpoint about these drugs.

It is clear that ERT will prevent many of the physical discomforts which may arise during menopause such as hot flashes, night sweats, vaginal dryness or atrophy, as well as preventing osteoporosis. Its effects on cardiovascular health are still unclear at this point. What ERT will not do is prevent wrinkles or outward signs of aging, nor will it help deal with the existential or psychosocial issues which menopause often

156

brings to the surface.

While proponents of ERT say that its use will increase life span by preventing hip and spinal fractures and cardiovascular disease, there are also drawbacks to ERT therapy. Side effects may include breast distention or soreness, water retention and edema, headaches, or mild to severe nausea. Severe side effects may include an increased risk for gallstones and gallbladder disease. Moreover, while studies linking the use of ERT to breast cancer are conflicting, most doctors will not prescribe it for women who have had breast cancer or who are at a high risk for that disease.

ERT is also not prescribed for women with clinical depression, uterine fibroids, diabetes, thrombophlebitis or other thrombo-embolic disorders, serious migraines, known gallbladder disease, nor is it usually prescribed for women who are overweight since women who are more than 25-30 pounds overweight are at a higher risk for uterine/endometrial cancer due to the fact that natural estrogen is formed in body fat tissue, and higher levels of blood estrogen have been linked to increased incidences of uterine cancer.

Finally, while some women feel much better on ERT, others dislike having a monthly "period". Still others find the increased visits to the doctor which ERT demands to be a financial strain. It is also true that increased visits to the doctor often result in more medical tests, more drugs, possibly even more surgeries.

## THE CHINESE MEDICAL VIEW

From the point of view of Chinese medicine, ERT, with or without progestins, has some definite drawbacks. These have

157

to do with 1) its potential side effects, and 2) the fact that if progestins are added it causes most woman to continue having a period, albeit a small one, for as long as they take it.

When looking at the potential side effects of ERT, one can see that they are similar to those of the birth control pill. This is not unusual, since both drugs contain estrogen, and in most cases, both contain progestin or progesterone as well. According to Chinese medicine, the way that the birth control pill causes infertility it by causing Blood Stagnation in the pelvis. Therefore, we might also suppose that ERT will do the same thing. Consider that unopposed estrogen can lead to uterine growths or exacerbate uterine fibroids, both of which, according to Chinese medicine are a species of Blood Stagnation. Blood Stagnation can cause a number of problems, the most immediate one being Qi Stagnation (See chart on p. 48), since the Qi and Blood flow together, and Stagnation of one will, over time, lead to Stagnation of the other. Since the smooth flow of Qi and Blood is largely controlled by the Liver, this Stagnation mostly affects the Liver, at least at first. Liver Qi Stagnation and its consequences have been discussed at some length in Chapter Four, but lets look at the possible side effect of ERT in this light.

Breast pain and distention are the first side effect listed. This symptom is always said to be due to Liver Qi Stagnation and consequent Heat and Congested Qi travelling through the Meridians which traverse the breast tissue. Nausea is caused by Liver Qi invading the Stomach which leads to the Stomach Qi rebelling up instead of descending as it must normally do. Edema or water retention is due to the Liver Qi adversely affecting the Spleen's ability to transport and transform Fluids. Headaches are another common sign of Liver Qi Congestion. In women headaches are usually a combination of Ascending

Liver Yang with Blood Deficiency. When the Liver Qi congests over a period of time, this Qi Congestion dries or exhausts the Blood. When the Congested Qi loses its root (Blood), it floats up or vents up, usually over the Meridian which traces the side or temporal region of the head, the Gallbladder Meridian. This causes neck and shoulder tension and pain, and headaches. Gallbladder disease is usually related to Damp Heat in the Liver and Gallbladder plus Liver Qi Congestion, and sometimes Blood Stagnation as well.

It is interesting also to note that many of the disorders which contraindicate the use of ERT, breast or uterine cancers, thromboembolic diseases, serious high blood pressure, severe migraines, uterine fibroids, stroke, and liver/gallbladder diseases, all typically involve either Liver Qi Stagnation, Blood Stagnation, or both. If ERT over a long period of time has a negative impact on these disorders, it is a logical hypothesis that ERT contributes to Liver Qi Stagnation and to Blood Stagnation.

In terms of the continued periods which women taking ERT experience, in Chapter Three on Chinese medical theories it was stated that after a certain point, the body recognizes that it can no longer support the continued loss of *Jing* Essence via the menstrual blood, and so, in its wisdom, the body stops the menstrual periods. It is possible from a Chinese energetic point of view that ERT is a *Jing* tonic which allows a woman to lose Blood each month without having a negative impact on her supply of either Pre or Post Natal *Jing*. If so, perhaps the loss of Blood each month is not the disaster that it first appears to be. If however, ERT does not in some way replace the *Jing* which would be lost each month with the shedding of the uterine lining, it would seem in the long run that this drug induced bleeding which the addition of progestin to ERT

159

brings about is not a good idea. However, without progestin, estrogen alone creates worse Blood Stasis, as demonstrated by the increased tendency to uterine neoplasms.

Whether ERT can be considered an effective *Jing* tonic is not clear at this point. In any case, it is clear that even if it does tonify *Jing*, it does not do so without side effects. This is not a very positive situation from the point of view of Chinese medicine.

## ERT ALTERNATIVES

We have, in the chapter on professional therapies, presented a number of herbal and orthomolecular alternatives to ERT which may be helpful for women who cannot or do not wish to take ERT. The Chinese medical rational and to some extent the Western nutritional rationale for these products has also been presented. The question remains however, on a biochemical level, as to how these various substances work, and whether they are effective because, especially in the case of herbs, they have naturally occurring estrogens and progestins in them.

In terms of vitamin/mineral substances the answer is no, they do not contain estrogen or progestins. What they do is to encourage the estrogen production of the adrenal glands, slow down estrogen inactivation by the liver, and encourage general metabolic, vascular, and endocrine balance and health. In the case of Metagenics' Fem-Estro™, the inclusion of Ginseng in the formula suggests that this herb is at least pro-estrogenic, which is to say it encourages estrogen production in the body. To be on the safe side Metagenics recommends that this formula should be contraindicated in cases such as breast cancer where excess estrogen is known to be a possible negative factor. As mentioned above, there has been only one reported case of side effects or problems with this supplement to date and this case did not involve breast problems at all[42].

Many herbs have been analyzed biochemically to find out exactly what substances they contain. It is known that some herbs do contain natural estrogens, or are at least pro-estrogenic in the body. That means that they encourage an increase in endogenous estrogen. From the point of view of Chinese medicine this may not be relevant, however, since the laws ruling the use of herbal substances and the monitoring of the outcome of that use have little to do with biochemistry. In Chinese medicine an herb or herbal formula is prescribed for a Chinese diagnosis, which does not include any mention of estrogen or other biochemical substances. The herbs are described as tonifying Yin or Yang, Qi or Blood, dispersing Stagnation, clearing Heat, or calming the Spirit, etc. If the use of an herbal formula alters the energetic balance in the body in such a way that the person's signs and symptoms are relieved without side effects or causing any long term problems, then the herbs can be said to have been safe and successful.

This is not to say that herbs are not medicine, that they cannot have side effects, or that some herbs may not have estrogen as part of their biochemical make-up. They are, they can, and some undoubtedly do. However, herbs properly administered according to a correct professional Chinese diagnosis do not have side effects even with long term use. Generally this is because, unlike synthesized drugs, an herbal formula is an energetically balanced combination of ingredients addressing more than one Organ, energy, or tissue in the body. This means that the substances in an herbal formula balance each other biochemically as well, making them easy for the body to absorb and metabolize without skewing the internal biochemistry wildly in any direction. Also, herbal and vitamin/mineral therapy work much more slowly and gently than Western drug therapy in general. In many cases one has to take herbs or vitamins for four to six weeks before major changes begin to be apparent.

For an example of how a specific formula might work in a balanced and holistic way in the body, let us describe Two Immortals from Health Concerns Co. which we discussed earlier. This formula has ingredients which tonify Blood, Yin, and *Jing* producing relief from such symptoms as night sweats and hot flashes. One might say that these herbs have a similar effect as estrogen does. These herbs are not given alone, however. They are balanced by ingredients which clear upwardly flaring Heat or harness Ascendant Liver Yang and reroot it in the pelvis where it belongs and where it is needed. This also prevents hot flashes, headaches, dry eyes, and irritability. Other ingredients tonify the Kidneys and bones, nourish the Sinews (Tendons) and Liver Blood. This encourages strength, stamina, flexibility, and proper bone density, and prevents musculoskeletal pain and stiffness. There are also ingredients which calm the Spirit and encourage proper sleep, drain Damp Heat and decongest the Liver and Gallbladder. This prevents liver or gallbladder disease. And finally, there are ingredients to invigorate the Blood and Qi to prevent problems related to Blood or Qi Stagnation. There are no known side effects to this formula if used based on a correct professional TCM diagnosis, nor is it linked to an increase in any other disease or disorder. It is easy to understand from this short description, then, how a well balanced herbal formula works in the body to reduce or eliminate uncomfortable symptoms, while at the same time balancing all the various functions and energies in the body without side effects. A single biochemical substance, such as is found in most Western

162

drugs, is incapable of such sophisticated, holistic balance.

## OTHER WESTERN THERAPIES FOR MENOPAUSAL COMPLAINTS

While ERT is the most common therapy used for menopausal and post menopausal women, there are other substances which are used in some situations. Androgens (male sex hormones) can be used for loss of sex drive and low energy. Thyroid hormones are sometimes used to good effect for women with low energy or wild energy swings. Diuretics are given for water retention and edema. Tranquilizers and sedatives are given for anxiety or sleep disturbances. All of these are helpful to some women, but all of them have possible side effects and all have the same drawback as was just described above. They are not a part of a balanced formula designed to work gently with the body as a whole. There are effective, non-iatrogenic Chinese herbal and orthomolecular remedies for all these accompanying signs and symptoms of menopause which work more gently and holistically to restore optimum balance to the body.

### SUMMING UP

What we know is that ERT and other hormonal therapies commonly used for menopausal complaints are effective at reducing or eliminating many symptoms. We also know that they all have potential side effects and possible unknown or unclear risks. In light of these unknowns, many women may wish to find alternative therapies that have a safer track record. This book is designed to inform women that such alternatives exist.

# APPENDIX II
# OSTEOPOROSIS: ALTERNATIVE
# TREATMENT OPTIONS

## OVERVIEW OF WESTERN TREATMENTS

Osteoporosis (OP) is considered to be a major health problem in America today affecting as many as 20 million Americans, 90% of which are post menopausal women. Approximately 50% of Caucasian women by the age of 75 will have spinal compression fractures.[43] The cost for treatment of osteoporosis in the U.S. is staggering and it is also associated with high mortality rates.

Primary OP is considered to have multiple causative factors including 1) failure to develop sufficient bone mass during youth, 2) excessive age related bone loss, 3) defective intestinal calcium absorption, 4) lowered blood estrogen levels beginning at menopause, and 5) sensitivity to parathyroid hormone calcitonin.[44]

For both preventive and remedial treatment of osteoporosis, Western medicine has many treatments. ERT is the primary one and is considered to be quite effective in preventing osteoporosis, but must be continued for life for continued protection. This is whether or not other symptoms indicating ERT use are present. (See Appendix I for information on ERT.) Other therapies include calcitonin, calcium carbonate supplementation, sodium fluoride, and a new drug called etidronate. Patients are also encouraged to get regular exercise of a weight bearing nature.

165

## Calcium Carbonate

This supplement is given in amounts of 2,400 to 3,600 milligrams per day. While it has the advantage of being very inexpensive, it is poorly absorbed by those with poor digestion because it causes an alkalinization of the stomach. Since hydrochloric acid (HCL) is necessary for the absorption of calcium in the intestine, an alkaline form of calcium is not really cost effective since it will not be as well absorbed, and it may cause further digestive difficulty by suppressing necessary HCL levels in the stomach. We will discuss other more effective sources of calcium below.

## Calcitonin

Calcitonin is a peptide hormone secreted by the parathyroid gland which inhibits the rate of calcium coming out of the bones into the bloodstream. It is available from human, pork, and fish sources and is sometimes administered singly, or in conjunction with ERT or sodium fluoride. Side effects from calcitonin therapy may include

## Sodium Fluoride

Fluorine (fluoride) increases the deposition of calcium in the bones, thereby increasing their strength. It is often used in conjunction with ERT, calcitonin therapy, or calcium supplementation in the form of sodium fluoride. Although traces of this mineral are beneficial to the body, excessive amounts are definitely harmful, inhibiting various enzyme processes which are vital to the metabolism of vitamins, causing calcification of ligaments and tendons, and even degenerative changes in the kidneys, liver, central nervous system, and heart. Sodium fluoride is found in drinking water supplies throughout the U.S.

today in order to prevent the decay of tooth enamel, although this form of fluorine is not the same as calcium fluoride which is how fluorine is found in nature. Sodium fluoride is toxic if it comprises more than two parts per million in water supplies. Women on long term sodium fluoride supplementation should have blood fluoride levels monitored regularly. It is interesting to note that calcium is a natural antidote to sodium fluoride poisoning. Seafoods, meat, cheeses, and certain types of tea are good sources of natural fluorine and, in general, fluorine deficiency is quite rare in the U.S.

### Etidronate

Etidronate works by inhibiting resorption of minerals by the blood from the bone. This is a new medicine for the treatment of osteoporosis and initial research studies with it are promising. Findings of a two year research study of 429 women with post menopausal OP conducted by the Massachusetts Medical Society concluded that intermittent cyclic etidronate therapy for 12 months resulted in significant increases in bone mineral density which were sustained for another 12 months after discontinuing use of the drug.[45] The improvement in bone mass mostly affected the spine, while other areas such as wrist and hip bones did not respond positively to this drug. Few side effects to this drug appeared in this study.

### ALTERNATIVE THERAPIES

While Western medicine has a number of therapeutic options for OP, it continues to be a major problem in post menopausal women in the U.S. as the statistics above indicate. In light of this, effective prevention and alternative therapies for this problem, especially ones which can be used safely over an extended period of time would be a welcome addition.

## Microcrystalline Hydroxyapatite (MCHC)

The most promising natural supplement for the treatment and prevention of osteoporosis is microcrystalline hydroxyapatite (MCHC). This is a whole bone extract that has been shown to improve calcium absorption. MCHC does not have the drawbacks of most calcium preparations because it is a compound containing the bone minerals calcium, phosphorus, magnesium, and fluoride in the normal physiological proportions. Not only has this substance been found to halt bone loss, but actually to restore bone mass in cases of OP.[46] It can be used both remedially and preventively, without side effects.

Metagenics, Inc. has two MCHC formulae. Cal-Apatite™ is an MCHC formula for people who are already taking a multivitamin/mineral supplement. Osteogenics™ is a more complete mineral formula designed for those who are not taking adequate minerals from any other source. Other companies may have similar formulas, and it is probably wise to consult a health practitioner before beginning any long term supplementation program.

### Herbal Remedies

As was stated earlier in this book, according to Chinese medicine, the bones are ruled by the Kidneys. Since aging largely involves the degeneration of the Kidneys, problems with bone loss, bone softening, arthritis, etc. are not surprising. The Chinese have largely treated aging problems with the bones, therefore, by tonifying Kidney *Jing*. There are a number of herbal formulas for doing this, many of which actually include varying amounts of bones. Unfortunately, some of these formulas call for the use of the bones of endangered animal species such as tigers or leopards. In light of this fact, I feel it is inappropriate to encourage the use of such formulas, although I have no doubt that they are effective. The use of synthesized bone compounds such as those listed above are a much more ecologically sound choice.

## OTHER PREVENTIVE MEASURES

It is well known that regular weight bearing exercise is crucial to the maintenance of bone mass. It is also important to know what activities or substances will deplete bone mass or speed up its loss. The list is not surprising, although some of us will be surprised/disappointed to know about all the things which we should avoid.

1. Excessive alcohol causes malabsorption of many vitamins and minerals including zinc, which is required for the synthesis of vitamin $D_3$, which is in turn required for bone mineralization.

2. Antacid products which contain aluminum (most over the counter products do). These increase the urinary and fecal excretion of calcium. Cooking with aluminum pots and pans has a similar effect. For people with hyperacidic digestive discomfort, there are other natural products on the market which will not cause this problem or other problems which may be related to aluminum ingestion. One such product is Metagenics Upper GI™.

3. Soft drinks, especially those with caffeine, cause significant increase in urinary calcium loss.[47]

4. Prolonged or repeated use of antibiotics, especially broad spectrum types, may directly affect calcium balance in the body. In a study by Lois Kramer and colleagues, it was noted that tetracycline use for three months induced significant increase in urinary calcium output and adversely affected collagen synthesis as well.[48]

5. Smoking accelerates bone loss as shown in studies comparing vertebral fracture levels in smokers and non-smokers.[49]

6. Caffeine. See #3 above. Everyone should know that caffeine is a poison, not a food. For an overview, see Chapter Eight on diet, page 107-108 of this book.

7. Excess phytic acid found in many unprocessed grains prevents the absorption of calcium into the bone. Grains which are partially processed, i.e., part of the bran is removed, are lower in phytic acid. This is interesting in light of the fact that in Chinese dietary theory, all grains should be at least partially processed for easier digestion. People who eat large amounts of bran should take higher amounts of calcium.

This list is not exhaustive. There are many other Western drugs and procedures which may affect bone mineralization including corticosteroids, dilantin, oral contraceptives, isoniazid, nystatin, hemodialysis, and gastric surgery.

Additionally, people with lactose intolerance, hyperthyroidism, or diabetes, are known to absorb minerals poorly or have insufficient amounts in their diet. Such people should supplement their diets with products such as Metagenics' Multi-Min Chelate, Osteogenics, and/or Cal-Apatite.

170

## SUMMING UP

Although osteoporosis and bone demineralization has undoubtedly been a problem for human beings for centuries, it is also probable that a sedentary lifestyle plus the increased consumption of caffeine, sugar, antibiotics, steroid drugs, aluminum-containing antacids, nicotine, and soft drinks seen in late 20th century America exacerbates the problem.  Along with preventive measures related to the above, people with high risk levels for OP would be well advised to supplement their diets with easily absorbable minerals, especially calcium. 90% of the people who experience OP in the U.S. are post menopausal women.  While Western drug intervention, especially ERT, is effective for preventing and treating OP, it appears that it can also be treated and prevented just as effectively through more natural methods which do not involve the possible risks of hormone therapy.

# ENDNOTES

1    Lyttleton, Jane, "Topics in Gynaecology Part One: Menopause", *Journal of Chinese Medicine*, Sussex, UK, #33, May, 1990, p. 5

2    Berkow, Robert, and Fletcher, Andrew, *The Merck Manual of Diagnosis and Therapy, 15th Edition*, Merck, Sharp, & Dohme Research Laboratories, Rahway, NJ, 1987, p. 1697

3    Ibid., p. 1713

4    McVeigh, Gloria, "Mastering Menopause: A Plan of Action for Every Symptoms and Side Effect", *Prevention Magazine*, Vol. 42, #4, April, 1990, p. 48

5    Ibid., p.48

6    Berkow, R., and Fletcher, A., op.cit., p. 1713

7    Ibid., p. 1714

8    Gambrell Jr., Don R., *Estrogen Replacement Therapy*, Second Edition, Essential Medical Information Systems, Inc., Dallas, TX, 1990, p. 29

9    Greenwood, Sadja, *Menopause Naturally, Preparing for the Second Half of Life*, Revised Edition, Volcano Press, Volcano, CA, 1989, p. 86

10   Gambrell, Don R., op.cit., p. 11

11   Berkow, R., and Fletcher, A., op.cit., p. 1075

12    I feel that more MD's are trying to provide their clients with information, both written and verbal, at a level which they can understand and which gives the client more personal power in their own healing process.

13    Kaptchuk, Ted, *The Web That Has No Weaver*, Congdon & Weed, NY, 1983, p. 35-36

14    Dr. Liang, as quoted in course notes, Dechen Yonten Dzo Institute of Buddhist Medicine, Feb., 1986

15    Wang, Tao-yang, "A Preliminary Discussion of the Bao Gong, Bao Mai, and Bao Luo", trans. by Zhang Ting-liang and Bob Flaws, *Blue Poppy Essays, 1988*, Blue Poppy Press, Boulder, CO, 1988, p. 17

16    Ibid., p. 18

17    Lyttleton, Jane, op.cit., p. 5

18    "Yang tends to be ever Excess, Yin tends to be ever Deficient." This statement is attributed to the great doctor of the Jin/Yuan Dynasty, Xu Dan-xi (1281-1358) and reflects the typical imbalance of Yin/Yang which he saw in most of his patients. Although Yin and Yang are a constant dynamic, their relatively balanced state is said to be approximately 2/5 Yin to 3/5 Yang.

19    *Chinese/English Terminology of Traditional Chinese Medicine*, Hunan Science & Technology Press, 1981, p. 10

20    Anon. "Build Exercise into Your Lifestyle", *Staying Well Newsletter*, American Chiropractic Assoc., May-June 1989, p. 1

21    Greenwood, Sadja, op.cit. p. 21

22    Gambrell, Don R., p. 22

23    Matsumoto, Kiiko, and Birch, Stephen, *Hara Diagnosis: Reflections on the Sea*, Paradigm Publications, Brookline, MA, 1988, p. 277-278

24    Ibid., p. 271-311

25    Flaws, Bob, "Pre-menstrual Breast Distention", *Free & Easy, Traditional Chinese Gynecology for American Women*, Second Edition, Blue Poppy Press, Boulder, CO, 1986, p. 104

26    Hsu, Hong-yen, and Preacher, William G., *Chen's History of Chinese Medical Science*, Oriental Healing Arts Institute, Long Beach, CA, 1977, p. 71

27    Lee, Miriam, *Clinical Applications of St. 36, Sp. 6, Co. 4 and 11, and Lu. 7: One Combination of Points Can Treat Many Diseases*, self-published, Palo Alto, CA, p. 70

28    Wolfe, Honora, *The Breast Connection: A Laywoman's Guide to the Treatment of Breast Disease by Chinese Medicine*, Blue Poppy Press, Boulder, CO, 1989. p. 74

29    Bland, Jeffrey, *Introductory Nutrition Course*, publisher and date unknown, p. 11

30    McLaren, H. G., "Vitamin E in Menopause", *British Medical Journal*, #17, Dec. 1949, p. 1378

31    Dunne, Lavon J., *Nutrition Almanac*, Third Edition, McGraw-Hill Publ. Co., New York, 1990, p. 226

32    Anon., "Vital Natural Vitamins", *Delicious Magazine*, Vol. 5, #1, Feb. 1989, p. 12

33    Anon. "Healthfront: Painful Breasts May Benefit From Iodine", *Prevention Magazine*, April, 1987, p. 12

34    Notes from Tuina Chinese Massage course at the Shanghai College of Traditional Chinese Medicine, May, 1986

35    Lyttleton, Jane, op.cit., p. 8

36    Bland, Jeffrey, op.cit., p. 11

37    Nutrition Masters Class notes, Metagenics, Inc.

38    Shoemaker, E.S., Forney, J.P., and MacDonald, P.C., "Estrogen Treatment of Postmenopausal Women: Benefits and Risks", *Journal of the American Medical Association*, #238, Jan., 1977, p. 1524

39    Greenwood, Sadja, op.cit., p. 90

40    "Report on Menopause", ABC network television, *20/20*, August 10, 1990

41    Gambrell, Don R., op.cit., p. 23

42    Oral reports on Fem Estro requested directly from Metagenics office.

43    Gambrell, Don. R., op. cit., p. 65

44    Berkow, R., and Fletcher, A., op.cit., p. 1296

45    Watts, Nelson B., et al., "Intermittent Cyclic Etidronate

Treatment of Postmenopausal Women with Osteoporosis", *The New England Journal of Medicine*, Vol. 323, #2, July 12, 1990, p. 73

46    Dixon, Allan St. J., "Non-hormonal Treatment of Osteoporosis", *British Medical Journal*, Vol 286, #6370, March, 1983, p. 999

47    Hollingberry, P.W., and Massey, L.K., "Effect of Dietary Caffeine and Sucrose on Urinary Calcium Excretion in Adolescents", Fed. Proc., #45, Abstract, 1986, p. 1286

48    Kramer, Lois, et al., "Drug-Mineral Interactions", Fed. Proc., Vol. 43, #4, Abstract, 1281, 1986, p. 375

49    Daniell, H.W., "Osteoporosis of the Slender Smoker: Vertebral Compression Fractures & Loss of Metacarpal Cortex in Relation to Postmenopausal Cigarette Smoking & Lack of Obesity", *Arch. Internal Medicine, #136, 1976, p. 398-404*

# SUGGESTED READING

## BOOKS ON WOMEN ISSUES AND MENOPAUSE

*Body Love - Learning to Like Our Looks & Ourselves,* Rita Friedman, PhD, Harper & Row, 1990.

*Menopause and The Years Ahead* by Mary K. Beard, MD.. & Lindsay Curtis, MD, Fisher Books, 1988. Supports the use of ERT therapy for most women.

*Menopause Naturally: Preparing for the Second Half of Life* by Sadja Greenwood, MD, Volcano Press, 1989. This book is a well rounded introduction to the Western medical ideas concerning menopause and the treatment of related complaints either with ERT or other more natural methods. Very well written.

*Prospering Woman - A Complete Guide to Achieving the Full Abundant Life* by Ruth Ross, PhD, Bantam New Age Books, 1989.

*The Goddess Within - A Guide to the Eternal Myths That Shape Women's Lives* by Jennifer Barker Woolger and Roger J. Woolger, Fawcett Columbine Books, 1989.

*The Menopause Self-Help Book* by Susan M. Lark, MD, Celestial Arts, 1990. Similar to Dr. Greenwood's book listed above, but with some good, specific exercise illustrations about stretching and yoga.

*Woman of a Certain Age: The Midlife Search for Self* by Lillian B. Rubin, Harper & Row, 1990.

*Women Coming of Age* by Jane Fonda with M. McCarthy, Simon & Schuster, 1984. This interesting, anecdotal book deals with many issues related to menopause and middle age.

## BOOKS ON CHINESE MEDICINE

*Chinese System of Food Cures - Prevention & Remedies* by Henry Lu, Sterling Publishing Co., 1986.

*Free & Easy - Traditional Chinese Gynecology for American Women* by Bob Flaws, Blue Poppy Press, 1986. A Chinese gynecology reference text with descriptions of many major gynecological problems and how they are described and treated by TCM.

*Hara Diagnosis: Reflections on the Sea* by Kiiko Matsumoto and Stephen Birch, Paradigm Publications, 1988. As mentioned in the chapter on self-help therapies, this book contains great detail concerning hara massage and hara diagnosis.

*Prince Wen Hui's Cook - Chinese Dietary Therapy* by Bob Flaws and Honora Lee Wolfe, Paradigm Publications, 1983. Chinese energetic description of over 150 foods, with many recipes for specific Chinese medical patterns of disharmony.

*The Breast Connection - A Laywoman's Guide to the Treatment of Breast Disease by Traditional Chinese Medicine* by Honora Lee Wolfe, Blue Poppy Press, 1989 Exactly as the title says, an introduction to Chinese medical theory as it pertains specifically to breast disease.

*The Web That Has No Weaver* by Ted Kaptchuk, Congdon & Weed, 1983 The best general introduction for anyone interested in exploring further Chinese medicine and its theories.

## BOOKS ON NUTRITION, EXERCISE, & RELAXATION

*Growing Younger - Nutritional Advice for Longevity, Vitality, & Health* by Gershon M. Lesser, MD, Jeremy Tarcher, Inc., 1990.

*Joy and Comfort Through Stretching & Relaxing* by Ursula Hodge Caster, The Seabury Press, 1982. For those who are

180

unable to do regular exercise.

*Nutrition Almanac* Third Edition, by Lavon J. Dunne. McGraw-Hill Publishers, 1990. This book presents detailed nutritional information on all micronutrients, dietary sources, and relevant research.

*Stretching* by Bob Anderson. Shelter Publications, 1980. This wonderful book includes stretching exercises for all parts of the body and specific stretches for participation in various sports.

*Stretch & Strengthen - A safe comprehensive exercise program to balance your muscle strength with lifelong flexibility*, by Judy Alter, Houghton Mifflin, Co., 1986.

*The Acupressure Stress Management Book - Acu Yoga* by Michael Reed Gach with Carolyn Marco, Japan Publications, Inc., 1981.

*The Chinese Exercise Book* by Zhou Dahong, MD, Hartley & Marks Publishers, 1984. From ancient and modern China - exercises for well-being and the treatment of illness.

*The Relaxation Response* by Herbert Benson, Avon, 1975. Ground breaking research on why relaxation therapy is important and how it works according to Western medical science.

*Yoga for a New Age - A Modern Approach to Hatha Yoga* by Bob Smith and Linda Boudreau Smith, Smith Productions, 1986.

# Index